Nocturia

Jeffrey P. Weiss · Jerry G. Blaivas
Philip E.V. Van Kerrebroeck · Alan J. Wein
Editors

Nocturia

Causes, Consequences
and Clinical Approaches

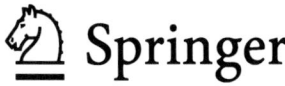

Editors
Jeffrey P. Weiss, MD, FACS
Department of Urology
SUNY Downstate College of Medicine
VA New York Harbor Healthcare System
Brooklyn, NY, USA
urojock@aol.com

Philip E.V. Van Kerrebroeck, MD,
PhD, MMSc
Department of Urology
University Hospital Maastricht
Maastricht, The Netherlands
kerrebroeck@urology.azm.nl

Jerry G. Blaivas, MD
Department of Urology
Weill Medical College of Cornell University
New York, NY, USA
SUNY Downstate College of Medicine
Brooklyn, NY, USA
jblvs@aol.com

Alan J. Wein, MD, PhD (hon)
Department of Urology
University of Pennsylvania
Philadelphia, PA, USA
alan.wein@uphs.upenn.edu

ISBN 978-1-4614-1155-0   e-ISBN 978-1-4614-1156-7
DOI 10.1007/978-1-4614-1156-7
Springer New York Dordrecht Heidelberg London

Library of Congress Control Number: 2011939061

© Springer Science+Business Media, LLC 2012
All rights reserved. This work may not be translated or copied in whole or in part without the written permission of the publisher (Springer Science+Business Media, LLC, 233 Spring Street, New York, NY 10013, USA), except for brief excerpts in connection with reviews or scholarly analysis. Use in connection with any form of information storage and retrieval, electronic adaptation, computer software, or by similar or dissimilar methodology now known or hereafter developed is forbidden.
The use in this publication of trade names, trademarks, service marks, and similar terms, even if they are not identified as such, is not to be taken as an expression of opinion as to whether or not they are subject to proprietary rights.
While the advice and information in this book are believed to be true and accurate at the date of going to press, neither the authors nor the editors nor the publisher can accept any legal responsibility for any errors or omissions that may be made. The publisher makes no warranty, express or implied, with respect to the material contained herein.

Printed on acid-free paper

Springer is part of Springer Science+Business Media (www.springer.com)

Dedications to
Nocturia: Causes, Consequences and Clinical Approaches

This book is dedicated to our families, patients, and residents who have inspired us to practice and teach medicine while advancing its knowledge.

We would also like to dedicate this textbook to Dr. Jens Peter Norgaard, who, with utmost academic integrity for the past two decades, has championed a most fruitful collaboration between academia and industry in advancement of the study of Nocturia.

Preface

Nocturia has been variously described as a symptom, a condition, a symptom complex, and a syndrome. A case can be made for any of these descriptions. By the simplest of criteria, nocturia is a symptom, defined below. However, a thorough understanding of the many medical and surgical conditions that may contribute to the genesis of nocturia in individual patients leads to the conclusion that diagnosis and treatment of this symptom are a gateway to high-quality medical care in the broadest sense. Physicians intent upon unlocking the many contributing factors to nocturia will find themselves learning amazing things about their patients, which most often rise well past the level of the lower urinary tract to include problems with cardiac, pulmonary, renal, endocrine, and nervous systems. It may well be that there is not another solitary symptom, the study of which ties together so much fascinating pathophysiology. It is for this reason that the editors devote an entire textbook to recording the state of the art in evaluating and managing this common and vexing medical complaint.

Brooklyn, NY	Jeffrey P. Weiss
New York, NY	Jerry G. Blaivas
Maastricht, The Netherlands	Philip E.V. Van Kerrebroeck
Philadelphia, PA	Alan J. Wein

Contents

1. **Introduction** 1
   Jeffrey P. Weiss

2. **Medical Conditions Associated with Nocturia** 11
   Emin Aydur and Roger Dmochowski

3. **Nocturia and Sleep Disorders: Morbidity, Mortality, Quality of Life and Economics** 37
   Sonia Ancoli-Israel, Donald L. Bliwise, and Jens Peter Nørgaard

4. **Diary-Based Population Analysis of Nocturia in Older Men: Findings of the Krimpen Study** 59
   Boris van Doorn and J.L.H. Ruud Bosch

5. **Epidemiology of Nocturia: Evaluation of Prevalence, Incidence, Impact and Risk Factors** 77
   Kari A.O. Tikkinen, Theodore M. Johnson II, and Rufus Cartwright

6. **Nocturia and Overactive Bladder** 109
   Jerry G. Blaivas and Johnson F. Tsui

7. **Nocturia and Surgical Treatment of the Prostate** 115
   David D. Thiel and Steven P. Petrou

8. **Lower Urinary Tract Pharmacotherapy for Nocturia** 127
   Roger Dmochowski and Alan J. Wein

9. **Nocturia and Antidiuretic Pharmacotherapy** 135
   Philip E.V. Van Kerrebroeck

10. **Nocturia in the Elderly** 147
    Catherine E. DuBeau and Johnson F. Tsui

11 **Nocturia: Treatment with Alternative Therapies** 157
    Duong D. Tu and Franklin C. Lowe

12 **Nocturia: Proposals for Future Investigation** 165
    Jeffrey P. Weiss

Index 169

Contributors

Sonia Ancoli-Israel, PhD Department of Psychiatry, University of California, San Diego, La Jolla, CA, USA

Emin Aydur, MD Department of Urology, Vanderbilt University Medical Center, Nashville, TN, USA

Jerry G. Blaivas, MD Department of Urology,
Weill Medical College of Cornell University, New York, NY, USA
SUNY Downstate College of Medicine, Brooklyn, NY, USA

Donald L. Bliwise, PhD Professor of Neurology, Psychiatry/Behavioral Sciences, and Nursing; Director, Program in Sleep, Aging and Chronobiology, Emory University School of Medicine, Wesley Woods Health Center, Atlanta, Georgia, USA

J.L.H. Ruud Bosch, MD, PhD Department of Urology,
University Medical Center Utrecht, Utrecht, The Netherlands

Rufus Cartwright, MRCOG, MD (Res) Queen Charlotte's
and Chelsea Hospital, Institute of Reproductive and Developmental Biology,
Du Cane Road, London, UK

Roger Dmochowski, MD, FACS Department of Urology,
Vanderbilt University Medical Center, Nashville, TN, USA

Catherine E. DuBeau, MD Division of Geriatric Medicine, University of Massachusetts Medical Center, Worcester, MA, USA

Theodore M. Johnson II, MD, MPH Emory University/Atlanta VA Medical Center, Geriatric Medicine and Gerontology, Atlanta, GA, USA

Franklin C. Lowe, MD, MPH Departments of Urology, Columbia University, College of Physicians & Surgeons and St Luke's/Roosevelt Hospital Center, New York, NY, USA

Department of Urology, New York Presbyterian Hospital – Columbia University Medical Center, New York, NY, USA

Jens Peter Nørgaard, MD, DMSc Medical Sciences Urology, Ferring International Pharmascience Center, Copenhagen, Denmark

Steven P. Petrou, MD Department of Urology, Mayo Clinic, Jacksonville, FL, USA

David D. Thiel, MD Department of Urology, Mayo Clinic, Jacksonville, FL, USA

Kari A.O. Tikkinen, MD, PhD Department of Urology and Department of Clinical Epidemiology and Biostatistics, Helsinki University Central Hospital, University of Helsinki, Helsinki, Finland

McMaster University, Hamilton, ON, Canada

Johnson F. Tsui, BS SUNY Downstate College of Medicine, Brooklyn, NY, USA

Duong D. Tu, MD Departments of Urology, Columbia University, College of Physicians & Surgeons and St Luke's/Roosevelt Hospital Center, Boston Children's Hospital, New York, NY, USA

Boris van Doorn, MD Department of Urology, University Medical Center Utrecht, Utrecht, The Netherlands

Philip E.V. Van Kerrebroeck, MD, PhD, MMSc Department of Urology, University Hospital Maastricht, Maastricht, The Netherlands

Alan J. Wein, MD, PhD (hon) Department of Urology, University of Pennsylvania, Philadelphia, PA, USA

Jeffrey P. Weiss, MD, FACS Department of Urology, SUNY Downstate College of Medicine, VA New York Harbor Healthcare System, Brooklyn, NY, USA

Chapter 1
Introduction

Jeffrey P. Weiss

Keywords Introduction • Nocturia • Nocturnal urine volume (NUV) • Nocturnal polyuria • Global polyuria • Mixed nocturia • Sleep Deprivation

Definition of Nocturia

Nocturia is defined by the International Continence Society as waking during the night at least once to urinate. It has additionally been suggested that a nocturia-related void is preceded and followed by sleep [1]. Whether sleep must follow a nocturia-related void is not entirely clear. Thus, for example, if someone arises an hour earlier than planned with the urge to void but could not return to sleep, nocturia seems evident but would not be considered as such if one rigidly adheres to the notion that a nocturia-related void must be followed by sleep. In the same sense, nocturnal voiding with failure to return to sleep leading to a second void which is then followed by sleep may cause confusion in designation of nocturia severity. Voiding during hours of sleep resulting from awakening for reasons other than the urge to void is not considered nocturia, although from a practical standpoint it is difficult to keep track of "convenience voids" at night as opposed to true nocturia-related voids. Thus, most studies of nocturia in the literature from a practical standpoint include voiding for all reasons during sleep hours.

There are several scientific questions associated with this definition. For example, how should sleep time be defined? Sleep time varies by individual but on average it is 8 h a night [2]. This definition can affect evaluation of nocturia as the number of nocturnal voids depends partly on how many hours an individual actually sleeps. Another question concerns whether the patient is awakened by the need to void or

---

J.P. Weiss, MD, FACS (✉)
Department of Urology, SUNY Downstate College of Medicine,
VA New York Harbor Healthcare System, Brooklyn, NY, USA
e-mail: urojock@aol.com

the patient voids after being awakened for other reasons. Although most patients in one study with nocturia were awakened by the need to void, the rest were awakened by thirst, uncomfortable temperature, noises, worry, pain or other stimuli [3]. Further, since at least 16% of the population is composed of shift workers who sleep during daylight, "nocturia" may in fact normally occur during the day [4].

Diary-Based Classification of Nocturia

Evaluation of nocturia begins with a focused history and physical examination with regard to aspects such as sleep quality, urinary complaints, fluid intake, cardiac problems, type and timing of various medications, prior lower urinary tract surgery and other comorbidities that might account for excessive nocturnal urine output, detrusor overactivity or abnormal bladder sensory function. A key tool in the evaluation and diagnosis of nocturia is the Frequency Volume Chart (FVC), in which patients record the volume and timing of daytime and nighttime voids for 1–3 days. The voiding patterns revealed by FVC data can provide clinicians with invaluable guidance regarding etiology and treatment. The use of FVCs is additionally recommended because of demonstrated discrepancies between nocturnal voiding data obtained using FVCs and data obtained from subjective questionnaires such as the International Prostate Symptom Score [5]. Based upon analysis of the 24 h FVC, the patient may be categorized as having any of the following: (1) nocturnal polyuria (NP); (2) low nocturnal bladder capacity despite normal global bladder capacity; (3) diminished global bladder capacity; (4) mixed (a combination of NP and low global or nocturnal bladder capacity) and (5) global (24 h) polyuria. Each category is associated with a differential of several medical conditions which may be investigated further and treated as part or all of the conditions associated with nocturia (see Table 1.1). Unfortunately, despite appropriate evaluation, in many patients clearly identifiable remediable conditions are not found, in which case nocturia may be idiopathic and would require a therapeutic approach on an empiric basis.

Nocturnal urine volume (NUV) is the volume of urine voided throughout the night, and includes the first morning void since this void is excreted by the kidneys during the hours of sleep. However, the first morning void is considered a normal diurnal voiding episode and should not be included with the tally of actual nightly voids. Maximum voided volume (MVV) is defined as the largest volume of urine voided throughout the 24-h period. The Nocturia index (Ni) is calculated by dividing NUV by MVV [6]. When the Ni is greater than 1 the NUV exceeds the bladder maximal storage capacity and nocturia occurs (enuresis may also occur if the patient does not awaken).

Nocturnal polyuria. NP is an increased production of urine at night which is offset by lowered daytime urine production such that 24-h urine volume remains within normal limits [7]. The nocturnal polyuria index (NPi) is defined as NUV divided by the 24-h urine volume. Normally, urine is produced in an age-dependent circadian pattern. In young people (age <25 years) mean $NPi = 0.14$ compared to that of older

Table 1.1 Diary-based categorization of nocturia and respective underlying medical conditions

Nocturia category	Underlying medical conditions
Nocturnal polyuria	• Congestive heart failure • Diabetes mellitus • Obstructive sleep apnea • Peripheral edema • Excessive nighttime fluid intake
Diminished global or low nocturnal bladder capacity	• Prostatic obstruction • Nocturnal detrusor overactivity • Neurogenic bladder • Cancer of bladder, prostate, or urethra • Learned voiding dysfunction • Anxiety disorders • Pharmacologic agents • Bladder, ureteral calculi
Global (24 h) polyuria	• Diabetes mellitus • Diabetes insipidus • Primary polydipsia

people (age >65 years) whose mean NPi = 0.34 [8]. Accordingly, the International Continence Society has defined NP to exist when 24-h urine production is within normal limits and NPi is greater than 0.33 [9]. Several other definitions of NP have been used. They include NUV greater than 6.4 ml/kg, nocturnal urine output >0.9 ml/min (54 ml/h) or higher [10] and >90 ml/h (see Chap. 4 below). Thus, for an "average" 70-kg person who sleeps about 8 h, the upper limit of urine excreted during the hours of sleep is expected to be from 450 to 720 ml, depending upon the cut point used. Diagnosis of NP leads to a differential diagnosis including excessive evening fluid intake (behavioral factors), third spacing (e.g., due to venous disease of the legs), cardiac dysfunction and obstructive sleep apnea [7–9].

Decreased nocturnal bladder capacity. The two types of nocturia due to diminished bladder capacity are (1) global decrease in bladder capacity as expressed by low MVV and (2) decreased nocturnal bladder capacity. In both conditions nocturnal urinary volume exceeds bladder capacity and the patient is awakened by the need to void because the bladder does not hold enough. Urological causes of low nocturnal and global bladder capacity include infravesical obstruction, idiopathic nocturnal detrusor overactivity, neurogenic bladder, cystitis, bladder calculi, ureteral calculi and neoplasms of the bladder, prostate or urethra. Urological evaluation for etiology of diminished NBC includes cystoscopic and urodynamic techniques for diagnosing these disorders. A useful means to evaluate the relationship between nocturnal voided volumes and the patient's own bladder capacity during a specific 24 hour interval is the nocturnal bladder capacity index (NBCi). NBCi is the actual number of nightly voids (ANV) minus the predicted number of nightly voids (PNV). PNV is derived by calculating the Ni (NUV÷MVV) and subtracting 1. NBCi is ANV−PNV. NBCi >0 indicates that nocturia occurs at volumes <MVV. As an illustration of the application of the NBCi, a patient who experiences nocturia six times

(ANV) and who voids 750 ml during the intended hours of sleep and has an MVV of 250 ml would have an Ni of 3. The PNV is the Ni−1, which in this case is equal to 2. Subtracting PNV from ANV results in an NBCi of 4, indicating a substantially diminished NBC. A significant association between patients with severe nocturia and NBCi >2 has been demonstrated [11] and a statistically validated cut point above which low nocturnal bladder capacity is associated with nocturia in a normative population is 1.3; therefore, urologic referral is recommended for these patients [12].

Timing of medication intake should be carefully sought during the history-taking interview. Certainly medications which pharmacologically decrease bladder capacity (e.g., beta blockers) may cause nocturia if taken just prior to retiring. While urological causes for low bladder capacity may be found, it is often difficult to distinguish resulting global from nocturnal decreases in bladder capacity. To some extent, therefore, treatment of low bladder capacity may benefit patients during the day and not night, or vice versa. Follow-up of such therapy is necessary in order to measure the benefit as specifically regards nocturia. Management of these disorders is discussed more fully in other articles in this textbook.

Mixed nocturia. Many patients with nocturia have a combination of NP and low nocturnal bladder capacity. An evaluation of 850 patients with overactive bladder revealed that diminished NBC plays a greater role in the pathogenesis of nocturia in younger patients, whereas in older patients NP assumes relatively greater importance [13]. In a study of 194 patients, nocturia was due to NP in 7%, low NBC in 57%, global polyuria in 23%, and a mixture of NP and low NBC in 36% [14]. In view of emerging evidence of the multifactorial etiology of nocturia in individual patients [15], the "mixed" category would seem to be particularly relevant, in that treatment yielding clinically satisfying outcomes will likely require institution of multiple incremental additive therapies. Verification of the latter statement mandates a considerable clinical research effort in the future.

Global polyuria. Polyuria is defined as a 24-h urine output greater than 40 ml/kg, causing daytime urinary frequency and nocturia occasioned by a general increase in urine output, outstripping even normal bladder capacity. This contrasts with NP in which 24-h urine volume remains normal but there is increased production of urine throughout the night. Inappropriate excretion of water in cases of polyuria leads to polydipsia to prevent circulatory collapse. Causes of global polyuria are diabetes mellitus, diabetes insipidus and primary polydipsia.

Uncontrolled diabetes mellitus leads to hyperglycemia and an osmotic diuresis predisposing patients to nocturia. Treatment for this etiology of nocturia is directed at decreasing the serum levels of glucose with diet, oral hypoglycemics and insulin where indicated.

Diabetes insipidus is a disorder of water balance. Central DI is caused by deficient synthesis of antidiuretic hormone secondary to loss of neurosecretory neurons in the hypothalamus or posterior hypophysis; nephrogenic DI is due to an inability of the kidneys to respond to ADH. When polyuria is demonstrated using the voiding diary, a water deprivation test may be performed to distinguish between DI and polydipsia [16].

Water deprivation testing involves the patient refraining from drinking throughout the night. If the patient usually drinks during the night the test should be done in a monitored setting to prevent dehydration. The first morning void is checked for osmolality. Osmolality greater than 800 mOsm/kg H_2O indicates both normal ADH secretion and normal renal response to ADH. Thus, a normal water deprivation test means that global polyuria is due to primary polydipsia. Primary polydipsia is either dipsogenic or psychogenic. Dipsogenic polydipsia is associated with a history of central neurological abnormality such as prior brain trauma, radiation or surgery. Psychogenic polydipsia is a long-term behavioral or psychiatric disorder.

If the water deprivation test is abnormal, a renal concentrating capacity test may be done to distinguish between central and nephrogenic DI. In adults 40 μg desmopressin is administered intranasally or 0.4 mg orally. The bladder is emptied and a urine sample for osmolality is obtained 3–5 h later. Water intake is restricted for the first 12 h after drug administration. The reference level for normal urine osmolality after desmopressin administration is greater than 800 mOsm/kg for most patients. If after an abnormal water deprivation test the renal concentrating capacity test is normal, the patient has central DI which can be treated with replacement doses of desmopressin. Considerably reduced concentrating capacity following desmopressin administration (urine osmolality <550 mOsm/kg) indicates nephrogenic diabetes insipidus. The latter may be due to chronic renal disease or the presence of conditions/medications blocking the action of ADH in the nephron. The latter may include lithium, tetracyclines, hypercalcemia and hypokalemia.

While the etiology of nocturia can be classified objectively by voiding diary analysis as described above, it cannot determine the degree of bother or consequences of nocturia in daily functioning. To enable physicians and researchers the opportunity to gather quantifiable information related by patients as to these subjective sequelae of nocturia and treatment outcomes, a number of patient-reported outcome (PRO) instruments have been formulated and validated. Among these include the Nocturia Quality-of-Life (NQoL) questionnaire, the International Consultation on Incontinence Questionnaire for Nocturia (ICIQ-N) and the Pittsburgh Sleep Quality Index (PSQI). The NQoL is a self-administered PRO instrument with evidence of validity specifically developed to assess the impact of nocturia and its treatment on patient's quality of life [17]. The ICIQ-N [18] is a brief self-administered instrument, summarizing the level of nocturia and its impact. It was created to help clinicians evaluate the symptom severity of daytime and nighttime voiding frequency, and the extent to which these symptoms bother patients with nocturia. The PSQI is a self-administered instrument that was specifically designed to measure sleep quality based on several components [19]. PSQI items were derived from clinician experience and a review of existing questionnaires on sleep quality. While the PSQI has not been specifically developed or validated for use in patients with nocturia, it has been shown to correlate with NQoL scores, demonstrating the relationship between the NQoL and PSQI regarding sleep impact of nocturia [17].

In addition to quantifying the degree and classification of nocturia through analysis of the FVC, consequences of nocturia in terms of bother, health-related quality of life issues and aspects of sleep degradation should be quantified with the use of selected patient reported questionnaires. FVCs and PROs may be repeated serially in order to both objectively and subjectively quantify the response to each intervention. Such baseline and follow-up evaluation is likely to be useful both in caring for individual patients, and to facilitate clinical research efforts designed to improve our ability to successfully intervene in populations afflicted with nocturia.

Consequences of Nocturia

Nocturia impacts multiple aspects of health including quality of life, health care costs, increased morbidity, missed diagnoses, and inappropriate treatment. Nocturia is associated with a great deal of stress, discomfort and functional impairment, an effect magnified in the elderly. Bother from nocturia is related to the frequency of episodes; in a population-based study, any degree of bother was associated with at least two episodes per night, and moderate to severe bother with three or more episodes [20]. Moderate-to-severe nocturia is associated with significant increase in both inpatient and outpatient health care costs, and number of hospitalization days [21]. Such costs are not limited to older adults. Nocturia may cause more sleep degradation and secondary sequelae such as mortality in younger people than that experienced by older adults [22, 23]. Whether caused or exacerbated by nocturia, these sleep interruptions may cause deterioration in the general health status. Such negative implications of nocturia may be particularly difficult for younger, working patients. Since younger adults are more commonly employed than elderly adults, nocturia in the more youthful working populace may occasion an economic impact significantly greater than in that of older individuals.

The impact of nocturia on work productivity was recently estimated using prevalence data from the Boston Area Community Health (BACH) Study and data from the US Bureau of Labor Statistics [24]. Subjects reporting nocturia had greater impairment in productivity as measured by the Work Productivity and Activity Impairment questionnaire (14% vs. 5%; 0%=maximum productivity, 100%=total loss of work productivity). The study concluded that the annual cost to US society resulting from loss of productivity from nocturia in the <65-year old population is approximately $61 billion per year, in addition to $1.5 billion per year for those ≥65 due primarily to the cost of treating complications of falls in the elderly.

Sleep Deprivation and Nocturia

In order to better appreciate the deleterious effects of nocturia, it is important to understand the effects of disrupted sleep. Sleep is a complex state consisting of non-rapid-eye-movement (NREM) sleep, typically subdivided into four stages, plus REM sleep. Diminished total sleep time correlates with increased daytime fatigue and decreased daytime alertness, both of which may increase the risk of falls, depressed mood, cognitive impairment and decreased quality of life, outcomes that are particularly relevant for older adults. Inadequate sleep duration accompanying nocturia is also associated with increased mortality [25]. Sleep deprivation (<6 h) has been associated with hypertension, obesity and glucose intolerance [26]. Population-based data have suggested that although insomnia is related to factors such as physical pain and depressed mood, nocturia represents an independent risk factor for compromised sleep quality [27].

Overview of Therapy of Nocturia

Outcome variables which may be useful in quantifying successful treatment of nocturia include: decreased episodes and/or bother from nocturia, increased time to first awakening, increased total daily sleep time, increased QoL, and diminished comorbidities. Assessment of outcomes of nocturia therapies should include an analysis of clinical vs. mere statistical significance: a significant treatment effect should be associated with a diminution in all the negative issues clinically associated with nocturia. Among available therapies for nocturia, most have no evidence-based medical (EBM) clinically significant studies (versus control) in their favor. These include: antimuscarinics [28–32], alpha adrenergic antagonists/5-alpha reductase inhibitors [33–36], combinations of antimuscarinics and alpha blockers [37], behavioral modification and serotonin/norepinephrine reuptake inhibitors. Transurethral prostatic resection (TURP) has had mixed results although generally TURP has benefited nocturia even when the benefit lags behind those of other lower urinary tract symptoms. In a 1986 article, 35% of patients prior to undergoing TURP had nocturia ≤2 whereas 3 years after TURP, 91% patients had nocturia ≤2 [38]. It is noted that in the latter non-randomized study, 24/84 (29%) of patients were lost to follow-up. On the other hand, Yoshimura in 2003 reported a non-randomized study demonstrating that among all seven questions on the IPSS, nocturia responded less well than the other LUTS questions [39]. However, the mean improvement in nocturia was a decrease in one episode nightly after TURP which competes well with all other known therapies for nocturia on an absolute basis. Cai et al. (2006) studied the International Consultation on Incontinence Nocturia Quality-of-life (NQoL) questionnaire in men undergoing TURP and found that the mean NQoL score improved significantly following outlet reducing surgery [40].

Antidiuretic therapy for nocturia can be utilized based upon EBM with an ICI grade 1-A and EAU 1b level of evidence/Grade A recommendation [41, 42]. The main potential side effect of such antidiuretic therapy as the peptide hormone desmopressin is hyponatremia, particularly experienced in the elderly, as well as in those with renal disease, cardiac disease and edema states. Non-peptide antidiuretic compounds in addition to desmopressin are being subject to investigation at the present time [43].

It is the hope of the editors of this textbook that the reader will develop confidence in his or her ability to evaluate and treat the many factors which may contribute to nocturia in individual patients. Methodology described herein will allow the practitioner to determine which if any of these treatments appear to be helpful both objectively (e.g., in terms of diminution in number of nocturic episodes, increase in sleep quality and quantity, improved effectiveness in the workplace and reduced mortality risks) and subjectively (e.g., in terms of effect on bothersomeness of nocturia). Such information should lead to future outcomes research allowing for development of evidence-based guidelines to best practices in management of patients with nocturia.

References

1. van Kerrebroeck P, Abrams P, Chaikin D, et al. The standardisation of terminology in nocturia: report from the Standardisation Sub-committee of the International Continence Society. Neurourol Urodyn. 2002;21:179.
2. Kripke DF, Garfinkel L, Wingard DL, et al. Mortality associated with sleep duration and insomnia. Arch Gen Psychiatry. 2002;59:131.
3. Bing MH, Moller LA, Jennum P, et al. Prevalence and bother of nocturia, and causes of sleep interruption in a Danish population of men and women aged 60–80 years. BJU Int. 2006; 98:599.
4. Beers T. Flexible schedules and shift work: replacing the '9-to-5' workday? Mon Labor Rev. 2000;23:33–40.
5. Blanker MH, Bohnen AM, Groeneveld FP, et al. Normal voiding patterns and determinants of increased diurnal and nocturnal voiding frequency in elderly men. J Urol. 2000;164:1201.
6. Weiss JP, Blaivas JG, Stember DS, et al. Evaluation of the etiology of nocturia in men: the nocturia and nocturnal bladder capacity indices. Neurourol Urodyn. 1999;18:559.
7. Asplund R. The nocturnal polyuria syndrome (NPS). Gen Pharmacol. 1995;26:1203.
8. Kirkland JL, Lye M, Levy DW, et al. Patterns of urine flow and electrolyte excretion in healthy elderly people. Br Med J. 1983;287:1665.
9. van Kerrebroeck P, Abrams P, Chaikin D, Donovan J, Fonda D, Jackson S, et al. The standardisation of terminology in nocturia: report from the standardisation sub-committee of the International Continence Society. Neurourol Urodyn. 2002;21:179–83.
10. Matthiesen TB, Rittig S, Norgaard JP, et al. Nocturnal polyuria and natriuresis in male patients with nocturia and lower urinary tract symptoms. J Urol. 1996;156:1292.
11. Weiss JP, Stember DS, Chaikin DC, Blaivas JG. Evaluation of the etiology of nocturia in men: the nocturia and nocturnal bladder capacity indices. Neurourol Urodyn. 1999;18:559–65.
12. Burton C, Parsons M, Weiss JP, Coats A. Reference values for the nocturnal bladder capacity index. Neurourol Urodyn. 2011;30:52–7.
13. Weiss JP, Blaivas JG, Jones M, et al. Age related pathogenesis of nocturia in patients with overactive bladder. J Urol. 2007;178:548.
14. Weiss JP, Blaivas JG, Stember DS, et al. Nocturia in adults: classification and etiology. Neurourol Urodyn. 1997;16:401.
15. Tikkinen KA, Auvinen A, Johnson 2nd TM, Weiss JP, Keränen T, Tiitinen A, et al. A systematic evaluation of factors associated with nocturia – the population-based FINNO study. Am J Epidemiol. 2009;170(3):361–8.
16. Adam P. Evaluation and management of diabetes insipidus. Am Fam Physician. 1997;55: 2146.
17. Abraham L, Hareendran A, Mills IW, Martin ML, Abrams P, Drake MJ, et al. Development and validation of a quality-of-life measure for men with nocturia. Urology. 2004;63(3): 481–6.

18. International Consultation on Incontinence modular Questionnaire (ICIQ). [online]. 2006. Available from: http://www.iciq.net/structure.html.
19. Buysse DJ, Reynolds III CF, Monk TH, Berman SR, Kupfer DJ. The Pittsburgh Sleep Quality Index: a new instrument for psychiatric practice and research. Psychiatry Res. 1989;28(2): 193–213.
20. Tikkinen KAO, Johnson TM, Tammela TL, et al. Nocturia frequency, bother and quality of life: how often is too often? A population-based study in Finland. Eur Urol. 2010;57(3): 488–96.
21. Nakagawa H, Niu K, Kaiho Y, Ikeda Y, Arai Y. Mortality in the elderly correlates with the frequency of nighttime voiding: results of a 5 year prospective cohort study in Japan. J Urol. 2010;183(4):e1–2.
22. Asplund R, Aberg H. Nocturnal micturition, sleep and well-being in women of ages 40–64 years. Maturitas. 1996;24(1–2):73–81.
23. Kupelian V, Fitzgerald MP, Kaplan SA, Norgaard JP, Chiu GR, Rosen RC. Association of nocturia and mortality: results from the Third National Health and Nutrition Examination Survey. J Urol. 2011;185(2):571–7.
24. Holm-Larsen T, Weiss JP, Langkilde LK. Economic burden of nocturia in the US adult population. J Urol. 2010;183(4):e1.
25. Ikehara S et al. Association of sleep duration with mortality from cardiovascular disease and other causes for Japanese men and women: the JACC study. Sleep. 2009;32(3):295–301.
26. Gangwisch JE, Heymsfield SB, Boden-Albala B, Buijs RM, Kreier F, Pickering TG, et al. Short sleep duration as a risk factor for hypertension: analyses of the first National Health and Nutrition Examination Survey. Hypertension. 2006;47(5):833–9.
27. Bliwise DL, Foley DJ, Vitiello MV, Ansari FP, Ancoli-Israel S, Walsh JK. Nocturia and disturbed sleep in the elderly. Sleep Med. 2009;10(5):540–8.
28. Cardozo L et al. Randomized, double-blind placebo controlled trial of the once daily antimuscarinic agent solifenacin succinate in patients with overactive bladder. J Urol. 2004;172: 1919–24.
29. Herschorn S, Swift S, Guan Z, Carlsson M, Morrow JD, Brodsky M, et al. Comparison of fesoterodine and tolterodine extended release for the treatment of overactive bladder: a head-to-head placebo-controlled trial. BJU Int. 2010;105(1):58–66.
30. Dmochowski R et al. Randomized, double-blind, placebo-controlled trial of flexible-dose fesoterodine in subjects with overactive bladder. Urology. 2010;75(1):62–8.
31. Brubaker L, Fitzgerald MP. Nocturnal polyuria and nocturia relief in patients treated with solifenacin for overactive bladder symptoms. Int Urogynecol J. 2007;18:737–41.
32. Rackley R, Weiss JP, Rovner ES, Wang JT, Guan Z. Nighttime dosing with tolterodine reduces bladder-related nocturnal micturitions in patients with overactive bladder and nocturia. Urology. 2006;67:731–6.
33. Koseoglu H et al. Nocturnal polyuria in patients with lower urinary tract symptoms and response to alpha-blocker therapy. Urology. 2006;67:1188–92.
34. Speakman M. Efficacy and safety of Tamsulosin OCAS. BJU Int. 2006;98 suppl 2:13–7.
35. Johnson-II TM, Jones K, Williford WO, Kutner MH, Issa MM, Lepor H. Changes in nocturia from medical treatment of benign prostatic hyperplasia: secondary analysis of the department of veterans affairs cooperative study trial. J Urol. 2003;170:145–8.
36. Johnson-II TM, Burrows PK, Kusek JW, Nyberg LM, Tenover JL, Lepor H, et al. The effect of doxazosin, finasteride and combination therapy on nocturia in men with benign prostatic hyperplasia. J Urol. 2007;178:2045–51.
37. Kaplan SA, Roehrborn CG, Rovner ES, Carlsson M, Bavendam T, Guan Z. Tolterodine and Tamsulosin for treatment of men with lower urinary tract symptoms and overactive bladder. A randomized controlled trial. JAMA. 2006;296:2319–28.
38. Bruskewitz RC, Larsen EH, Madsen PO, Dorflinger T. 3-year follow-up of urinary symptoms after transurethral resection of the prostate. J Urol. 1986;136:613.
39. Yoshimura K et al. Nocturia and benign prostatic hyperplasia. Urology. 2003;61:786–90.

40. Cai T et al. Impact of surgical treatment on nocturia in men with benign prostatic obstruction. BJU Int. 2006;98:799–805.
41. Oelke M, Bachmann A, Descazeaud M, et al. Guidelines on conservative treatment of non-neurogenic male LUTS. EAU; 2010 http://www.uroweb.org/gls/pdf/BPH%202010.pdf.
42. Andersson K-E et al. The pharmacological treatment of nocturia. BJU Int. 2002;90 Suppl 3:25–7.
43. Weiss JP, Yea C, Nathadwarawala M, Marks BK, Imnadze M. Novel non-peptide pharmacologic therapy for nocturia in men. J Urol. 2010;183(4):e590.

Chapter 2
Medical Conditions Associated with Nocturia

Emin Aydur and Roger Dmochowski

Keywords Nocturia • Age • Gender • Ethnicity • Polyuria • Lower urinary tract • Sleep • Socioeconomic • Reproductive • Lifestyle

Background

Nocturia had traditionally been considered part of an array of symptoms of some other primary disorder [1]. In 2002, the standardization subcommittee of the International Continence Society (ICS) proposed the first standardization of nocturia terminology and this report has marked a new era in the approach to the management of nocturia. Since then, nocturia has begun to be recognized as a clinical entity in its own right rather than a symptom of some other disorder, or classed as one of many lower urinary tract symptoms (LUTS) [2]. Although this proposal based on reasonable theoretical considerations has not been tested in any research and should not be taken as the result of scientific enquiry [3], approximately 100 research studies have cited the report within 8 years after its publication. Thus, the report plays a fundamental role of conceptual framework for research on nocturia to understand the possible causative or contributing factors to the pathophysiology of this entity, as the current knowledge on nocturia needs improving in order to advance clinical care.

There are good epidemiological data from worldwide, showing nocturia is a common condition that affects both men and women to an equal extent [4]. The bother experienced by patients with nocturia as well as the impact on quality of life, daytime functioning, and overall health can be severe. Therefore, it is important for the causes of nocturia to be diagnosed accurately so that effective treatment can be

E. Aydur, MD • R. Dmochowski, MD, FACS (✉)
Department of Urology, Vanderbilt University Medical Center, Nashville, TN, USA
e-mail: roger.dmochowski@vanderbilt.edu

given as necessary [1]. However, the current knowledge on factors associated with nocturia is limited. Studies of the pathophysiology of nocturia have generally been small and highly focused on one aspect of potential underlying causes [5].

Nocturia is a complex and highly multifactorial condition. According to the ICS report, nocturia can be related to one or a combination of three primary underlying causes, all of which increase with age: bladder storage problems, usually as a component of overactive bladder syndrome (OAB), detrusor overactivity (DO), urgency urinary incontinence, or bladder outlet obstruction (BOO) in men; 24-h polyuria; nocturnal polyuria (NP) as a frequent but often overlooked cause [2]. However, nocturia may be associated with many possible risk factors and comorbidities, such as snoring, obesity, prostate cancer, or restless legs syndrome [4]. These associations may not preclude specific causation, and most are certainly at least potentially contributory to the symptom. While an association between these risk factors and nocturia has been established, estimates of the proportion of patients with nocturia who are in fact affected by each underlying factor are less common in the literature [1]. Factors underlying nocturia may differ between individual patients, but may also coexist within one patient. It is therefore crucial that clinicians and other healthcare providers are well informed as to the characteristic "fingerprints" of each etiological factor, so that they can make treatment decisions which maximize the potential to achieve benefits for the patient [6].

The multifactorial nature of this condition is best demonstrated by the recent findings of the FINNO study which systematically assessed factors related to nocturia in a large population based survey [4]. The factors with the greatest impact for the population were urgency of urination, benign prostatic hyperplasia (BPH), and sleep disruption as manifested by snoring in men. In women, urgency, obesity, and snoring were predictive. Other associations included history of prostate cancer and antidepressant use in men, and coronary artery disease and diabetes in women. In another, multi-institutional study, 60% of subjects had daytime lower urinary tract symptoms (LUTS); one third had cardiac disease and 7% peripheral edema. NP was the most important contributor to nocturia [7]. Finally, it may be necessary to setup multidisciplinary teams to assess patients with nocturia to include urologists, gynecologists, cardiologists, endocrinologists, nephrologists, geriatricians, sleep specialists, as well as allied healthcare professionals such as physiotherapists and nurses [3].

This chapter specifically focuses on what is known about the predictive and risk factors for nocturia. In this chapter, risk factor is used as an aspect of personal behavior or lifestyle, environmental exposure, or inborn or inherited characteristic, which, on the basis of epidemiologic evidence, is known to be associated with nocturia considered important to prevent, while predictive factor means a condition or finding that can be used to help predict whether a patient with nocturia will respond to a specific treatment. Predictive factor may also describe something that increases a person's risk of developing nocturia. From the point of view of public health, it is important to identify the risk factors for nocturia that might impair the quality of life of the sufferers. This will allow for the provision of lifestyle behavior modification in patients at risk or for treatment of the underlying risk factors, which will be helpful in preventing and treating nocturia [8].

Demographic Factors (Age, Gender, and Ethnicity)

The ICS has defined nocturia as the number of voids recorded during a night's sleep: each void is preceded and followed by sleep [2]. Thus, the term nocturia, in contrast to the definition commonly used before 2002 (≥2 nocturnal voids) is not restricted to any particular number of nocturnal voids [9]. Moreover, this definition has excluded predefined thresholds and terms like "bother" and "complaint" because their use could result in a distortion of the determination of incidence, prevalence, course, and risk factors and therefore, this new term is considered a good definition for use in epidemiology studies [10].

Although a substantive association between age and nocturia has been established in several epidemiological studies, nocturia is an underreported condition and, therefore, the true extent of the problem in the population may be underestimated [1]. Adult patients are more likely to consult a provider if they have three or more episodes [11]. Nocturics may be embarrassed or reluctant to discuss their problems [1]. Moreover, they perceive nocturia to be a natural part of aging and therefore may fail to seek medical assistance or may not realize that treatment is available [12].

Several reports of nocturia prevalence exist in the literature. Although Irwin et al. have reported half of all adults to experience nocturia [13], the prevalence rates for nocturia vary considerably, and are affected by the population studied, the definition of nocturia used as stated earlier and the age range considered. For example, some studies investigated nocturia in a population exclusively at specific age groups. This may cause overall rates to be misleading [1]. For instance, Zhang et al. report a prevalence of only 9% in their random sample of Chinese women 20 years old or older. However, 84% of their sample was in fact younger than 50 years and, therefore, the relatively low overall prevalence may be influenced by the predominance of younger participants [14]. Despite these variations in the prevalence of nocturia, there are some findings which are reported repeatedly across studies and countries, when factors such as definitions of nocturia and age of the sample population are consistent [1]. On the other hand, Asplund and Aberg conducted one of the best studies showing prevalence variation due to the definition used for nocturia. They demonstrated a large difference between the incidence of one nocturnal voiding episode ($\cong 50\%$) and two ($\cong 10\%$) or three ($\cong 5\%$) episodes in a questionnaire survey of 3,669 randomly selected women aged 40–64 years in Sweden to assess nocturnal micturition patterns [15].

Bosch and Weiss have recently reported their literature review of 45 studies published in between 1990 and 2009 relating to the prevalence of nocturia in a population sample. They found that 20–44% of women in their 20s and 30s reported experiencing at least one void per night while 4–18% of women in this age category reported two or more voids nightly. Of women in their 70s and 80s, 74–77% reported one or more voids per night while 28–62% reported two or more voids nightly. Of men in their 20s and 30s, 11–35% reported at least one void per night while 2–17% reported two or more voids nightly. Of men in their 70s and 80s, 69–93% reported at least one void per night while 29–59% reported at least two voids per night.

Based on their findings, they concluded that all studies showed a tendency for nocturia to increase with age for both genders [1]. Also, typical ranges for ≥2 nocturia episodes/night has been reported as 5–15% for those aged 20–50 years, 20–30% for those aged 50–70 years, and 10–50% for those aged ≥70 years [10].

On the other hand, severity of nocturia increases with advanced age, even though more severe nocturia is less common than less severe nocturia. The majority of older men and women experience at least one void per night and on average up to two-thirds experience two or more voids per night. Around half of the population experiences at least one void per night from the age of 50 to 60 years while approximately 25% of the population experiences two or more voids nightly by their early 60s [1].

Descriptive epidemiological data indicate that the prevalence of nocturia increases with age, regardless of the definition used and the steepest increase is in older groups (>65 years) [10]. There are several studies reporting prevalence rates of two or more voids approaching or exceeding 50% in older populations [16] and being as high as 90% for one episode per night in persons over age 80. This increasing prevalence highlights the pervasive nature of this underreported condition [1]. In older age groups, nocturia has been variably associated with chronic medical conditions such as hypertension and diabetes, advancing renal failure, and cardiovascular disease. Nocturia in the frail elderly can cause accidental falls. Frail elderly persons with nocturia, who also have gait and balance disorders and other risk factors for falls, are clearly at increased risk for injury and consequent morbidity. Also, nocturia makes adult patients "feel old" and worry about falling at night [5].

It is well established that nocturia is associated with aging. In general, the incidence and severity of nocturia increases consistently from early adolescence to senescence [10]. However, it is not solely a feature of aging [17]. This increasing prevalence is largely due to age-related physiological changes [18] or pathological conditions that underlie the pathophysiology of nocturia, such as low bladder capacity, NP, or sleep disorders [5]. It is evident that an increase in nighttime urine excretion, causing individuals to rise and void, is part of the normal aging process. Interplay between physiological changes in renal conserving ability and hormonal systems regulating water and sodium handling alters the diurnal rhythm of nocturnal diuresis. These physiological and pathological changes associated with aging explain why NP is believed to contribute to at least 50–65% of cases of nocturia [12]. Finally, with advancing age more time is spent in bed and there are more nighttime awakenings to void. Nocturia can be considered as both a disease and as part of normal association of plasma arginine vasopressin and aging; it is the relative contribution of each of these factors that remains to be clarified [19].

A substantial proportion of younger adults are also affected. In practical terms up to one in five or six younger people consistently wake to void at least twice each night on average. The negative impact of sleep fragmentation caused by nocturia may be particularly difficult for these younger patients because they are more likely to have active lifestyles and demanding work schedules.

There are no large differences in the prevalence of nocturia between men and women; however, voiding at least once nightly tended to be reported more frequently in younger women than in younger men (20–44% and 11–35%, respectively), but is equally common or more so in men in older age groups [1], particularly after age 60 [5].

Interestingly, Tikkinen et al. reported that young women are more than 10 times more likely to have nocturia than young men in the Finnish population [20]. However, there are several studies reporting a similar rate of nocturia in men and women across all age groups [21, 22]. The reasons for the possible increased prevalence of nocturia in younger women versus men, and/or factors relating to study design which may lead to these varied findings, are subjects for further investigation. It may be that women experience greater fragmentation of sleep due to other causes (e.g., child care at night) or that they are simply more prone to insomnia than men and that these issues affect the reporting of nocturia. It is interesting to note that the studies that do indicate a gender difference in younger people come from several different countries and continents (Europe, Asia, Australia, and Canada). Therefore, the underlying reasons for this observation are unlikely to be confined to a specific country or culture [1].

Van Dijk et al. suggested that women start to develop nocturia at a younger age than do men, based upon their findings in a population-based survey designed to estimate the prevalence of nocturia in a representative sample of the adult population in the Netherlands [23].

In men, nocturia has been noted to be more significantly correlated with age than with bladder outlet obstructive symptomatology [24]. In another assessment of an elderly male population, 33% of 2,934 men had nocturia (greater than two episodes per night). However, multivariate analysis revealed the contributions of other pathologies to the symptom of nocturia including cerebrovascular disease, lower urinary tract (LUT) cancer, alcohol consumption, and treatment for voiding disorders [25].

The prevalence of nocturia, as with many other conditions, may be different among ethnic or cultural groups [19]. In fact, disparities in racial and ethnic presentations of nocturia have also been reported by several authors. Kupelian et al., in the BACH study, a large prospective assessment of a community-based population, identified an overall nocturia prevalence of 28.4% with higher prevalence rates in blacks (38.6%) and Hispanics (30.7%) as compared to white participants (23.2%) regardless of gender [26]. Similar findings have been observed by Sarma et al. in a study examining associations between diabetes and clinical markers of BPH in community-dwelling white and black men aged 40–79 years: black men had an increased association between irritative LUTS and diabetes [27]. However, Platz et al. reported that older black men were not more likely to have LUTS than were older white men with an apparent modestly higher prevalence of LUTS in older Mexican-American men [28]. Chuang and Kuo investigated the prevalence of LUTS, including nocturia, among indigenous and nonindigenous women in Eastern Taiwan and observed indigenous women have a higher prevalence of nocturia than nonindigenous women [29]. In a prospective comparison study, Mariappan et al. reported that nocturia, nocturia indices, and variables from frequency–volume charts are significantly different in Asian and Caucasian men with LUTS and they concluded that there are also possible ethnic differences in the causes of nocturia, with NP being more prevalent in Caucasians [30].

Table 2.1 Lower urinary tract factors associated with nocturia

Physiological change associated with aging (e.g., urogenital atrophy caused by estrogen deficiency)
Infravesical obstruction
• Bladder outlet obstruction (BOO)
• Urethral stenosis/urethral stricture
Nocturnal detrusor overactivity
• Idiopathic (OAB)
• Neurogenic (e.g., multiple sclerosis)
Detrusor hyperactivity with impaired contractility
Learned voiding dysfunction
Anxiety disorders
Pharmacological agents
Urinary stone disease (Ureteral calculi, bladder calculi)
Cystitis: bacterial, interstitial, tuberculosis, radiation
Cancer of the bladder, prostate, or urethra
Painful bladder syndrome/interstitial cystitis
Bladder hypersensitivity
Excessive nocturnal fluid input
Extrinsic compression (uterine fibroids, urogenital prolapse, ovarian tumor)
LUT surgery

Lower Urinary Tract Factors

Nocturia is the most prevalent of LUTS in the general community, as common in women as it is in men. Nocturia is also reported to be one of the most bothersome of LUTS, with greatest impact on the patient's quality of life. Although the ICS report highlighted for the first time the unique nature of nocturia as a LUTS that can arise purely due to disorders outside the LUT, and recent researches have confirmed this phenomenon, it is clear that many LUT factors (Table 2.1) affect bladder function during both daytime and nighttime, such as age-related changes in LUT, BOO, OAB, and cystitis. Disorders such as reduced absolute bladder capacity due to radiation are unlikely to change. In contrast, functional disorders that affect storage capacity may indeed be altered as people lie down and/or enter different sleep stages. Little research has been done to explore the possible effects of position, sleep, and/or hypnotic medications on bladder function in health and disease [6].

Nocturia has been noted to occur in association with LUTS such as incontinence. Massolt et al. noted that 48% of incontinent women experienced nocturia which was due to either NP with or without changes in functional bladder capacity in 75% of 111 women undergoing assessment [31]. Klingler et al. identified the different factors contributing to nocturia in 324 patients in a multi-institutional study. Mean nocturia was 2.8 in men versus in 3.1 women. Fifty percent of patients were aged >65 years, 60% had daytime LUTS as well as nocturia. Principal causes for nocturia were global polyuria in 17%, NP in 33%, and reduced functional capacity <250 ml in 16.2%; 21.2% had mixed forms of NP and reduced bladder capacity and 12.6% suffered from other causes. Quality of life was significantly lower in women, in patients aged >65 years and in those with reduced functional capacity. They concluded that nocturia had a high impact on bother score, strong associations with poor health, and other LUTS [7].

Age-related changes in the LUT may cause nocturia with or without other conditions such as NP or other LUTS. Detrusor contraction strength declines with age in women as well as men, and there is no DO-associated increase in contractility [5]. The alteration in collagen-to-smooth muscle ratio seen in later life leads to a "stiffer" bladder, with a lower elastic limit and may result in a reduction in functional bladder capacity and reduced sensation of bladder filling and thus LUTS, including nocturia [17].

Estrogen deficiency in postmenopausal women results in structural and physiologic changes, including urogenital atrophy, pelvic organ prolapse, pelvic floor relaxation, and neurogenic detrusor hyperactivity. Consequently, these alterations cause irritative symptoms and nocturia [18].

Age-related prostate epithelial hyperplasia is mediated by numerous stromal factors. It remains unclear whether prostatic inflammation (acute or chronic) contributes to urinary retention and LUTS in men [16].

Finally, both structural and functional changes occur with aging in the urinary tract and may increase the risk for development of nocturia, by decreasing bladder capacity and thus, nocturnal voided volume in both genders. In addition to the age-associated physiological changes to LUT function in later life, the elderly with nocturia appear to have a higher 24-h urine production than age-matched controls with no nocturia. These individuals also produce a higher proportion of their daily urine output at night [17]. Kawauchi et al. studied the role of reduced voided volumes in the elderly and analyzed nocturnal urinary frequency, time of voiding, and amount of each void in 188 healthy men (mean age 67.1 years) with no prostatic disease. Nocturnal urinary frequency increased with age from a mean of 0.61 voids per night at 55–59 years to 1.2 at 75–79 years. However, multiple regression analysis showed that nocturnal voided volumes and nocturnal urinary volume were independent determinants of nocturnal frequency; age was not an independent factor [32].

Diminished bladder capacity refers to a condition in which voiding occurs at bladder volumes less than functional bladder capacity, leading to awakening to void at night. Reduction in bladder capacity can occur at all times (reduced global bladder capacity) or exclusively at night (reduced nocturnal bladder capacity). Diminished global capacity is often related to urologic conditions, including BOO or decreased detrusor contractility resulting in increased postvoid residual urine volume (PVR), bladder irritation from stones, infection or neoplasm, extrinsic bladder compression from ovarian cancer or uterine fibroids, and decreased bladder capacity because of urogenital aging. BPH and OAB are two main urologic conditions associated with diminished bladder capacity [18] and just as there is a tendency to presume that nocturia in women is attributable to OAB, there is also a propensity for clinicians to attribute nocturia in men to prostatic problems, which can obstruct the bladder outlet and cause LUTS [6].

Among men with difficulty in emptying their bladder because of prostate enlargement, there is increased occurrence of LUTS, including nocturia. Nocturia and other

LUTS resulting from BOO are commonly associated with DO or high postvoid residuals. However, Chang et al. evaluated the cause of nocturia in a study of men and found that 83% had NP, 20% had NP alone, and 63% of patients had NP in combination with another factor such as small nocturnal bladder capacity, BOO, or sleep apnea [33]. Crucially, therefore, most male nocturia patients have NP, with or without comorbid prostatic problems. Men seeking help with their urinary problems are most frequently prescribed a1-adrenoceptor antagonists and 5 alpha-reductase inhibitors or a combination of these. The impact of these drugs on relief of symptoms of BOO has been well demonstrated, but less information is available on how these treatments affect increased nocturnal frequency. A beneficial effect of terazosin and to a lesser extent, finasteride, has been shown. However, most of alpha receptor antagonists interfere with blood pressure regulation and have a potential to cause postural hypotension. More selective a1-AR antagonists have a reduced propensity to cause this adverse effect [17]. On the other hand, failure of traditional therapies for BOO often is attributable to the presence of underlying NP: Yoong et al. report that 85% of BPO patients with nocturia unresponsive to alpha1-blocker treatment have NP [34]. Surgery (TURP) and traditional pharmacological therapies for BPO therefore frequently fail to provide a significant reduction in nighttime voiding [35, 36]. However, in the VA Cooperative Study Program Trial conducted by Johnson et al., 1,078 men with BPH having baseline nocturia of 2.5 episodes per night were randomized to receive empirical treatment with terazosin, finasteride, terazosin, and finasteride combined, or placebo. Nocturia episodes decreased to around two per night for all groups. No significant difference was found among any of the treatment arms, including placebo, suggesting that nocturia in men with BPH results from factors besides BOO [37].

Prevalence of the overactive bladder syndrome (OABS) increases in association with late life and is the a common cause of LUTS in the elderly. Nocturia commonly occurs as a result of this. Especially around menopause many women experience LUTS, including nocturia because of reduced endogenous estrogen production. Already existing symptoms often become worse when women enter menopause and if not treated, the condition further deteriorates [38]. When considering the symptom complex that constitutes the OABS, it is interesting to note that, in a European physician survey, nocturia was identified by only 5% of 355 physicians as the most important LUTS to resolve. However, 37% of those physicians identified it as the most difficult to deal with [17]. Weiss et al. studied 129 women ranging in age from 17 to 94 years. Of these 8% had NP, 62% had nocturnal DO, and 30% had a mixed form. Therefore, 32% must have had nocturia because of detrusor overactivity and no NP [39]. Brubaker and Fitzgerald report that, in the 62% of their OAB patients who had NP, solifenacin monotherapy led to no significant improvement in nocturia compared with placebo [40].

Increased urinary frequency may occur as a result of uninhibited detrusor contractions in neurological conditions such as a dementia, stroke, Parkinson's disease, and multiple sclerosis [19]. Urinary symptoms in patients with multiple sclerosis are usually secondary to spinal lesions, which interrupt neural pathways connecting the pontine micturition center to the sacral micturition center resulting in DO, small bladder capacity, and nocturia [41]. Another interesting urodynamic observation particularly in elderly people is detrusor hyperactivity and impaired contractile function. It may present as urinary retention and thereby mimic prostatic outlet obstruction. Resnick et al. reported 33% of institutionalized incontinent elderly people to have this abnormality [42].

A range of urological and gynecological diseases such as UTI, BPH, radiation cystitis, interstitial cystitis, and cancer and estrogen deficiency may also increase nocturnal urinary frequency, usually by decreasing bladder capacity [19].

Medical (nonurological) causes of reduced voided volumes are exemplified by factors such as medications and anxiety disorders, and can usually be discerned from patient history [43].

Diuretics have been associated with a doubling in nocturia in both men and women; this may be partly because most patients take these oral medications in the morning [9]. In a study by Reynard et al., diuretics taken 6 h before going to bed resulted in substantially less nocturia [44]. In contrast to these results, a recent study by Rembratt et al. found no significant correlation between nocturia and diuretic use, when diuretics were presumably used for heart failure/hypertension [45]. The occurrence of ≥ 3 nocturnal voids was reportedly three times higher in women using analgesics daily than in those not using analgesics [9].

Cardiovascular

Nocturia can be caused by cardiovascular diseases, including congestive heart failure (CHF), coronary artery disease, hypertension, lower extremity venous stasis disease through third-spacing of fluid in the lower extremities, and cerebrovascular events such as stroke.

Several studies have also shown nocturia to be associated with cardiovascular disease. Klingler et al. identified the different factors contributing to nocturia in a multi-institutional study of 324 patients. Nocturia and its associated problems were evaluated using Kings' Health Questionnaires and voiding diaries in conjunction with concurrent health variables. Sixty percent of subjects had daytime LUTS as well as nocturia, one third had cardiac disease, 33% had cardiac pathologies, and 7% peripheral edema. NP was the most important contributor to nocturia [7]. In addition to several factors, the BACH study identified cardiac disease especially when associated with increased BMI as increasing the risk of nocturia [46]. In a case-control study with prevalence sampling, Tikkinen et al. explored the correlates for nocturia and their population-level impact in subjects (aged 18–79 years) from the Finnish Population Register. Although numerous correlates were identified, none affected $\geq 50\%$ of nocturia cases of both sexes. However, they found that coronary artery disease was associated with nocturia in the age-adjusted analyses for both sexes but for only women in multivariate analysis [4]. In the analysis by Coyne et al. of responses from 5,204 adults participating in the National Overactive Bladder Evaluation survey, a diagnosis of CHF was found as a risk factor for nocturia [21].

In a survey of adults at ages 60 years or greater, Johnson et al. found that hypertension was a significant predictor of nocturia more than once nightly [47]. Gourova et al. investigated the prevalence of nocturia and the predictive relationships with several factors, including cerebrovascular disease, cardiovascular disease, hypertension, and others in 2,934 elderly men. The prevalence of nocturia (two or more nocturnal voids) was 32.9%. They determined that nocturia in elderly men was significantly related to cerebrovascular disease. Also, BPH had a significant relationship with nocturia, especially in respondents with hypertension. Cardiovascular disease or hypertension was significantly related to nocturia, mutually replacing each other as a risk factor [25]. However, epidemiological researches of the association between nocturia and cardiovascular disease are not always in agreement and some studies have not found cardiovascular disease a correlate for nocturia [22, 48–50]. Finally, although the association between nocturia and cardiovascular diseases is clear, it may be crudely extrapolated that these conditions are relatively modestly increased in patients presenting with nocturia compared with levels in the background population. The majority of patients with nocturia in the related studies were not affected by these conditions. Therefore, the key causes of nocturia for most patients encountered in clinical practice are likely related to other factors [1] and this supports the conclusion that cardiac diseases are not the most common causes of NP in nocturics, particularly in the elderly [51].

CHF, especially in incompletely treated cases and right-sided disease, leads to NP as a result of an increase in the atrial natriuretic peptide (ANP) [52]. ANP is an important factor in controlling sodium excretion through its direct natriuretic effect, and suppression of renin and aldosterone secretion. With advanced age, the basal ANP level has been shown to be three to fivefold higher than those of young adults. Additionally, plasma rennin and aldosterone activities are also decreased with aging. Further, in patients with edema-forming states such as CHF or venous system dysfunction in the lower extremities, large quantities of fluid and solute accumulated in the lower extremities while standing during the day may become mobilized into the circulatory systems at night when the patient is supine [18, 51]. Torimoto et al. evaluated 34 men with NP using bioimpedance analysis, and identified correlations between nocturnal volumes and extracellular fluid and leg volume changes indicating a re-centralization phenomenon in at least some individuals with NP [53]. Consequently, atria are distended with the mobilized fluid in CHF and therefore, atrial pressure increases [50]. ANP is released by atrial myocytes in response to atrial distension and sympathetic stimulation. With the aforementioned hormonal changes, ANP affects the kidneys by increasing GFR and filtration fraction, which in turn produces natriuresis and diuresis [18] and nocturia is therefore common in persons with edema in the legs of various origin such as CHF and lower extremity venous dysfunction. On the other hand, circulating vasopressin can increase markedly in proportion to the severity of cardiac failure. NP in this disease cannot therefore be explained by impairment of the vasopressin system [51]. It was recommended that "considerable caution" be exercised in prescribing exogenous AVP (desmopressin or DDAVP) to patients with cardiovascular disease or hypertension, and DDAVP should not be used in frail elderly with nocturia because of the exaggerated risk of hyponatremia [5, 54].

Hypertension has previously been shown to be associated with NP and nocturia [55]. Hypertension might be related to nocturia by its effect on cardiovascular physiology (edema, CHF with atrial stretch, and release of ANP) or renal physiology (renal effects on glomerular filtration and tubular transport). Hypertension may cause resetting of the pressure natriuresis relation in the kidney [47]. Recently, Agarwal and colleagues have noted associations of nocturia with nondipping (failure to lower blood pressure during night and sleep) and effects on hypertension [56].

On the other hand, there is substantial evidence of an independent association between obstructive sleep apnea (OSA), nocturia, and cardiovascular disease, which is particularly in the case of hypertension and stroke (refer to Chapter 3) [57].

Short and fragmented sleep has been linked with an increased risk of cardiovascular disease, traumatic injury because of a combination of postural hypotension resulting in impaired balance and nocturnal awakenings for frequent visits to the toilet and urgency, and possibly mortality [14, 18]. Asplund reported that older people who voided three or more times at night had been reported to have a greater mortality over a 54-month period. Heart disease and autonomic dysfunction may be responsible for this increased risk [58]. Also, elderly people with disrupted sleep patterns have mortality rates due to cardiac disease, stroke, cancer, and suicide at least 1.5 times higher than those of elderly people who do not suffer from interrupted sleep [12].

Cardiovascular events are clustered in the morning hours, after increases in blood pressure and heart rate that accompany awakening and arising. Similar hemodynamic changes occur during the night after nocturnal awakening and getting up. Such changes are common among older patients who have nocturia frequently and rise to urinate. Bursztyn et al. tested the hypothesis that nocturia >2 times at night may be associated with increased mortality in a population sample of 456 subjects born from 1920 to 1921. Twelve-year survival was significantly lower among subjects reporting nocturia compared with those without nocturia. The interaction between nocturia and previous coronary heart disease (CHD) was highly significant. Survival of patients who had CHD with nocturia versus those without nocturia was 44% versus 66%. They concluded that nocturia is a significant independent predictor of mortality among 70-year-old patients with known CHD and thus warrants special attention [59].

Pulmonary

Patients with chronic obstructive pulmonary disease (COPD; bronchial asthma and pulmonary emphysema) have an increased airway resistance with related NP possibly due to increased renal sodium and water excretion mediated by raised concentrations of ANP [60]. Although the association between nocturia and lung disease has not yet been fully elucidated, the study conducted by Bing et al. is unique to show an independent association between nocturia and lung disease for the first time in a population-based study. They evaluated the association between nocturia and several factors, including lung disease in a questionnaire study of 2,799 men and women and found lung disease was independently associated with nocturia and the association was strongly dependent on severity of nocturia, even though the study population diminished with advancing age. The authors postulated that the mechanism might be related to hemodynamic changes. Distension of the atria, acute hypoxia, and pulmonary hypertension has been reported to be responsible for an increase in ANP levels., leading to increased natriuresis and diuresis, which may play a role in the increase of nocturia episodes seen in these patients, though they stated that they did not know whether the similar mechanisms occur in patients with lung disease [50].

Also, Tikkinen et al. conducted a population-based study of 6,000 adults aged 18 to 79 years in Finland, studying nocturia and bother and health-related quality of life (HRQoL). They report that HRQoL worsens in proportion to an increase in the number of voids per night. In this study, nocturia was also associated with other comorbidities such as OSA and obstructive lung disease that also affect HRQoL [61]. Again, in a retrospective study, Oztura et al. demonstrated a significant association between nocturia and sleep disordered breathing, respiratory disturbance, sleep apnea–hypoxia, and low oxygen saturation [62]. However, Yosihimura et al. rejected an independent association between COPD and nocturia (≥2 voids) in their study [22].

Sleep-Related Factors (See Also Chap. 3)

Nocturia is a frequently described symptom that may be associated with a variety of sleep disorders [63], including insomnia, obstructive or central apnea syndrome, snoring, periodic or restless leg syndrome, parasomnias, sleep disorders related to medical disease, such as COPD, and sleep disorders related to neurological disease, such as Alzheimer's or Parkinson's disease and stroke [2] (Table 2.2). Sleep disturbance may be a cause or consequence of nocturia and these disorders causing nocturia may be related to concomitant medical or psychiatric conditions [64].

Sleep disorders are common particularly in the elderly and those are frequently the source of awakenings from sleep. The high incidence of both nocturia and sleep disorders in the elderly and other patients suggests that sleep disorders may be the cause of awakenings from sleep rather than nocturia [38]. Pressman et al. reported only 5% of his patients to correctly identify the source of their awakening from sleep. Most of awakenings from sleep attributed by the patients to be due to pressure to urinate were instead a result of sleep disorder [65].

The prevalence of nocturia in sleep disorders has not been extensively studied, even in OSA [63]. In an earlier study of women aged 40–64 years, Asplund and Aberg found that frequent nocturnal micturition was associated with poor sleep, daytime sleepiness, and impaired well-being [15]. In a home sleep study, the prevalence of OSA was double among urogynecology patients with nocturia compared with those without [66]. Klingler et al. reported that of NP patients with nocturia,

Table 2.2 Sleep-related factors leading to nocturia

Insomnia
Obstructive or central apnea syndrome
Snoring
Periodic limb movement disorders (periodic or restless leg syndrome)
Parasomnias
Sleep disorders related to medical disease (COPD, heart diseases, endocrine disorders such as thyrotoxicosis, acromegaly, rheumatoid arthritis, osteoarthritis, etc.)
Medications (corticosteroids, diuretics, β-adrenergic antagonists, calcium channel blockers, selective serotonin reuptake inhibitor antidepressants)
Sleep disorders related to psychiatric conditions (depression, anxiety, consumption and withdrawal of alcohol)
Sleep disorders related to neurological disease (Alzheimer's disease, Parkinson's disease, stroke, nocturnal epileptic seizures, dementia)

2.3% had sleep apnea [7]. Umlauf et al. reported nocturia to be closely associated with OSA in community dwelling older men and women [67]. Moriyama et al. found the prevalence of nocturia was high among patients with OSA and that OSA might have some relationship to nocturia without other voiding symptoms in men less than 50 years of age [68].

Nocturia has been reported to be an independent predictor of both self-reported insomnia and reduced sleep quality [69]. Yoshimura et al. investigated the differences and associations between bothersome (BN) and nonbothersome nocturia (NBN) and sleep disorders including insomnia, OSA restless leg syndrome (RLS), and periodic limb movement disorder (PLMD). Insomnia and OSA closely correlated with both NBN and BN, and PLMD correlated with BN. However, RLS was not associated with either NBN or BN [70].

Snoring has been associated with nocturia [71]. Oztura et al. reported that the prevalence of nocturia was 52% in individuals with primary snoring, 57.2% in individuals with mild OSA, 64.3% in individuals with moderate OSA, and 76.9% in individuals with severe OSA [62]. Gopal et al. reported that nocturia was associated with sleep disorders including OSA and insomnia in perimenopausal women [72]. Older African Americans have been reported to have twice the rates of sleep apnea of Caucasians, while a significant association between episodes of nocturia and symptoms of OSA was reported in African-American women [73, 74].

Nocturia is particularly bothersome for patients and their partners due to sleep disturbance [7]. The clinical implications of nocturia are naturally dependent on age and mobility, and on how often one has to get up during the night together with the ability to go back to sleep after returning to bed. Some have major sleep disturbances because of impaired sleep quality and daytime fatigue leading to lack of concentration [38].

However, deep, slow-wave, restorative sleep occurs during the first hours of the night, and lighter (less restorative) sleep predominates in the second part of the night. On the basis of the findings that it is mainly a decrease in deep sleep that contributes to daytime fatigue, researchers speculated that waking during deep sleep would also be more likely to leave patients feeling groggy and tired the next day. Therefore, the quality of sleep and quality of life are affected not only by nighttime voiding frequency, but also by the timing of waking to void [75].

With increasing numbers of nocturnal voiding episodes, women are also more prone to experience poor appetite, unhappiness, and lack of confidence in the future. In addition, they paid more visits to doctors and received more medical treatment. The number of days on the sick list was five times higher in women with three or more voiding episodes than in those without nocturnal voiding [15].

OSA is manifested with symptoms of poor sleep quality, daytime sleepiness, snoring, and nocturnal leg movements. Nocturia is an independent predictor of severe OSA in patients with ischemic stroke. Severe OSA increases the risk of stroke recurrence and mortality after stroke [76]. Similarly, a recent retrospective study found that sleep-disordered breathing symptoms in poststroke subjects were associated with more episodes of nocturia [77].

The mechanisms for the association between OSA and nocturia severity might be multifactorial. NP is found in most nocturics and may be secondary to factors such as aging, stroke, and OSA [76].

Fluid Volume Disturbance

Fluid volume disturbance can be caused by several reasons and results in either global polyuria or NP as frequent causes of nocturia [2, 7, 60].

Global polyuria is defined as urine production in excess of 40 mL/kg of body weight over a 24-h period [2]. Physiologically, the rate of urine production is controlled by two factors: the concentration of urine and the rate of solute excretion. The former is determined by the antidiuretic hormone, arginine vasopressin (AVP), which acts upon connecting tubules and collecting ducts within the nephron via activation of V2 receptors to increase the amount of water reabsorbed from the glomerular filtrate. The latter is composed mostly of urea, sodium, and potassium whose rate of excretion is determined by diet and other factors influencing protein metabolism and the extracellular fluid volume [64]. Global polyuria has been linked to DM (type 1 and type 2) with associated osmotic diuresis; to the condition diabetes insipidus (DI) with its associated deficient production of antidiuretic hormone by the posterior pituitary (central DI) and resultant polydipsia and polyuria; and to conditions that impair the ability of the kidneys to respond to antidiuretic hormone (nephrogenic DI) (Table 2.3). Among these, the link between DI and global polyuria is the only association that is well supported by research, with documentation that treatment of DI results in resolution of polyuria [3]. In addition, global polyuria may be due to primary polydipsia (excessive fluid intake) which is distinguished from DI by water deprivation testing [18]. Patients with primary polydipsia can concentrate urine to 600–800 mOsm/kg whereas those with DI cannot. Patients with DI can be further substratified to central or nephrogenic via ability to concentrate urine caused by exogenously administered desmopressin, an ADH congener, in

Table 2.3 Causes of global polyuria

Osmotic diuresis
- Poorly controlled diabetes mellitus (Type 1 or Type 2)
- Medications (e.g., mannitol, sorbitol)

Water diuresis
- Diabetes insipidus (DI)
    - Central (hypothalamic or pituitary lesions)
    - Renal (e.g., lithium, iatrogenic, hypercalcemia, hypokalemia, tetracyclines, hereditary, polyuric renal failure)
    - Gestational
- Primary polydipsia
    - Psychogenic
    - Dipsogenic

patients with central DI. Primary polydipsia can be either psychogenic, characterized by aggressive water consumption due to psychological and cognitive impairment, or dipsogenic, caused by a primary abnormality in the thirst mechanism in the setting of a structural brain abnormality [64].

Nocturnal urine volume is defined as the total volume of urine passed during the night (including the first morning void). Healthy young adults between the age of 21 and 35 years old excrete $14 \pm 4\%$ of their total urine volume between 23:00 and 07:00 h whereas the more elderly people excrete $34 \pm 15\%$. Clearly, while many of the patients with polyuria may also have NP, there are other conditions which may present with nocturia. These may be summarized as those that cause a water diuresis alone and those that cause a combined solute and water diuresis [64]. NP is an overproduction of urine at night (defined as urinary output greater than 20% of the daily total in young individuals and greater than 33% in older individuals), which is offset by lowered daytime urine production resulting in normal 24-h urine volume [2, 43]. A state of altered hemodynamics is an important factor in the etiology of NP in patients with edema-forming states, such as CHF, hypoalbuminemia, nephrotic syndrome, venous insufficiency, and CKD. Enhanced ANP secretion because of medical conditions such as OSA can also cause NP. ANP is released by atrial myocytes in response to atrial distension and sympathetic stimulation. As stated previously, it affects the kidneys by increasing GFR and filtration fraction, which in turn produces natriuresis and diuresis. Theoretically, sleep deprivation can also change hemodynamics and thereby increase nighttime urine production, adding to the complexity of the relationship between sleep and nocturia. Moreover, there is some indication that nocturia can be resolved with treatment of OSA [1, 18]. The assertion by review articles that NP is linked to excessive evening fluid intake, evening caffeine intake, CHF with associated edema, autonomic dysfunction, kidney disorders, or central neurologic disorders is reasonable, but not supported by research that delineates the pathophysiology of these associations and/or the normalization of voiding patterns with treatment of the underlying problem. Without this supporting evidence, it remains a possibility that the clinical association is obscuring one or more other, perhaps more important contributors [3] (Table 2.4).

Table 2.4 Factors leading to nocturnal polyuria

Water diuresis
Abnormality in nocturnal secretion (or action) of AVP (nocturnal polyuria syndrome)
Primary – Idiopathic
Secondary – Behavioral factors (e.g., excessive fluid intake shortly before retiring, late-evening diuretic intake)
Solute/water diuresis
Edema-forming states (e.g., CHF, CKD, nephrotic syndrome, hypoalbuminemia, hepatic failure, chronic liver disease, venous insufficiency)
Comorbidities (e.g., autonomic nervous system dysfunction, Alzheimer's disease, multisystem atrophy, stroke, Parkinsonism)
Sleep disordered breathing and sleep apnea syndrome
Renal failure
Estrogen deficiency

NP is often missed during the evaluation and diagnosis of nocturia despite the fact that it is perhaps the most common factor underlying nocturia [1]. Of men with LUTS suggestive of BPO, up to 95% may have NP [78]. Therefore, those patients will have no improvement even if they are given medical or surgical therapy for BOO.

Socioeconomic Factors

Socioeconomic factors have been associated with nocturia in a few recent reports, including marital status, education, employment, household income, and urbanization. However, the association is inconsistent among these studies. In the Boston Area Community Health (BACH) Survey conducted by Kupelian et al., the prevalence rates of nocturia by race/ethnicity and the contribution of socioeconomic status (SES) to potential differences by race/ethnicity were investigated in a random sample of 5,501 adults (2,301 men, 3,200 women) age 30–79. Nocturia was defined as voiding more than once per night in the past week or voiding more than once per night fairly often, usually, or almost always in the past month. Self-reported race/ethnicity was defined as black, Hispanic, or white. SES was defined as a combination of education and household income and categorized as low (lower 25% of the distribution of the SES index), middle (middle 50% of the distribution), and high (upper 25% of the distribution). They found that the effect of SES (education plus income) was more pronounced among men and among hispanic participants, while differences in prevalence of nocturia remained significant for black men and women. It was concluded that SES accounts for part of the race/ethnic disparities in prevalence of nocturia [26].

Burgio et al. studied the prevalence and correlates of nocturia (≥ 2 per night) in 1,000 community-dwelling older adults (aged 65–106) among whom African-American women, African-American men, white women, and white men were equally distributed. In-person interviews included social information (education, Mini-Mental State Examination, and rural versus urban dwelling). Nocturia was more common in men than in women and more common in African Americans than whites. Higher Mini-Mental State Examination score was protective in men and a higher education was protective for women, while they did not report any effect of urbanization on nocturia [73]. However, Johnson et al. reported that restricting the sample to those with a high school education or greater made little substantive difference in the correlations between nocturia and the educational status in a population-based, community sample of noninstitutional adults aged 60 and older, initially collected in 1983 in the Medical, Epidemiologic, and Social aspects of Aging (MESA) Study [47].

In a study conducted by Hsieh et al., a total of 3,537 women aged 20–59 were interviewed face to face, assessing risk factors for nocturia among Taiwanese women aged 20–59 years. Marriage was found to increase the risk of nocturia in women [8].

Tikkinen et al. explored the correlates for nocturia and their population-level impact in a survey of 3,579 male and female subjects (aged 18–79 years) randomly identified from the Finnish Population Register (62.4% participated; 53.7% were female). Questionnaires also contained items on sociodemographic factors (marital status, education, employment, urbanization). They did not report a correlation between nocturia and any of these socioeconomic factors [4].

Female Reproductive/Gynecologic Factors

In women, LUTS including nocturia are often believed to result from aging, childbirth, menopause, or just "being a woman" [60, 79]. In fact, it is known that incontinence in women increases with the number of childbirths and the frequency of urogenital symptoms increases at ages around the menopause [15]. The LUT is known to be estrogen sensitive; reduced endogenous estrogen production at menopause may explain the increased incidence of urinary symptoms during menopause. Systemic estrogen replacement therapy appears to alleviate some of these symptoms [38].

Lack of estrogen contributes to ultrastructural changes of impaired contractility (e.g., detrusor fibrosis) in women, while low estrogen also may contribute to bladder muscle cell differentiation. In the urethra, closure pressure decreases by an estimated 15 cm H_2O per decade, possibly related to mucosal changes extending to the bladder trigone, irritating sensory afferent nerves, triggering DO, and both decreased urethral vascular density and blood flow. Circular smooth muscle mass and fiber counts decrease, with striated muscle loss in the anterior urethra. There is evidence for denervation in uterosacral ligaments and levator muscles, and decreased muscle fiber number, type, and diameter. Moreover, pelvic floor dysfunction, such as pelvic laxity has been postulated as a cause of nocturia, as well other LUTS [80]. Postmenopausal atrophy may cause loss of lactobacillus and colonization with pathogenic organisms (*E. coli*, enterococci), leading to higher rates of bacteriuria and symptomatic urinary tract infections [16] which contribute to nocturia as well as other LUTS.

Asplund and Aberg analyzed the relationship between nocturnal micturition and gynecological factors such as parity, menstrual status, menopausal symptoms, and hormone replacement therapy in 3,669 Swedish women aged 40–64 years. Of women with no nocturnal micturition, 13% were receiving HRT, whereas the corresponding proportions in women treated HRT having one, two, and three or more nocturnal voiding episodes were 21, 23, and 28%, respectively. The number of nocturnal voiding episodes was unaffected by parity. The absence of an increase in nocturia in women of this study after several childbirths may support the view that nocturia can also be caused by other factors than disturbances in the distal urinary tract [15].

Tikkinen et al. evaluated the association of nocturia and urinary urgency with reproductive factors, including parity, the postpartum period, menopause, hormone replacement therapy, hysterectomy, and surgery for stress urinary incontinence (SUI) in randomly selected 2,002 women aged 18–79 years. Parity, postpartum (defined as 6 weeks to 1 year after delivery) and postmenopausal periods were associated with increased nocturia, but hormone therapy and hysterectomy were not. These authors found nocturia to be associated with parity when assessed independently of menopausal status [81].

Hsieh et al. analyzed the relationship between nocturia and some gynecological factors in 3,537 Taiwanese women aged 20–59 years and found that there was no relationship between nocturia and parity, menopause or hormone therapy. Although the women who underwent hysterectomies had a higher rate of nocturia than those who did not, the difference was not statistically significant [8]. Bing et al. reported no association between nocturia and parity, hysterectomy, pelvic organ prolapse, or urinary incontinence surgeries [50]. Similarly, Burgio et al. found history of HRT and hysterectomy to be unassociated with nocturia [73].

Lifestyle and Behavioral Factors

Many epidemiological studies have implicated lifestyle and behavioral factors to increase the risk for nocturia. These factors include body mass index (BMI) and obesity, fluid intake particularly at night, smoking and physical activity. Shiri et al. investigated the effects of lifestyle factors such as obesity, smoking, alcohol and coffee consumption on the incidence of nocturia in a sample of 1,580 men and found obesity to increase the risk of nocturia. The link between other lifestyle factors and nocturia is weak for alcohol consumption and absent for both smoking and coffee consumption [82].

There are potentially modifiable risk factors for nocturia in adults. Recently, Soda et al. conducted a prospective evaluation of 56 patients treated at three hospitals between 2005 and 2009 for symptomatic nocturia to test the efficacy of nondrug lifestyle measures as a first step in treating nocturia and found factors predictive of the efficacy of the intervention. Lifestyle modifications consisted of four directives of (1) restriction of fluid intake, (2) refraining from excess hours in bed, (3) moderate daily exercise, and (4) keeping warm in bed. The frequency volume chart, International Prostate Symptom Score, and Pittsburgh Sleep Quality Index before and 4 weeks after the intervention were used to evaluate the efficacy of therapy. The authors reported that mean nocturnal voids and nocturnal urine volume decreased significantly from 3.6 to 2.7 and from 923 to 768 ml, respectively. Fifty-three percent improved by more than one episode. They concluded nondrug lifestyle measures to be effective in decreasing the number of nocturia episodes and to improve quality of life. Patients with polyuria had a better response to this regime [83].

On the other hand, Nakagawa et al. reported a significantly increased mortality risk for nocturics (≥ 2 voids per night) compared with those people who experienced <2 voids per night. This risk was independent of many possible contributing comorbidities or lifestyle factors such as BMI, smoking and alcohol consumption, possibly due to fragmentation of sleep itself, and the health consequences of poor sleep [84, 85].

BMI and Obesity

Several epidemiological studies have consistently reported higher BMI or obesity as an important risk factor for nocturia, although the exact mechanism by which obesity causes nocturia is not known [86]. However, it confers increased risk for sleep apnea that is frequently associated with nocturia [43].

Tikkinen et al. analyzed the association of nocturia with overweight and obesity in over 3,500 randomly selected Finns aged 18–79 years. Self-reported body weight and height were used to calculate BMI. Subjects were classified on the basis of BMI as nonoverweight (BMI<25), overweight (BMI 25–29.9 kgm^2), or obese (BMI>or=30). Among men, the age-standardized prevalence of nocturia, defined as at least one void per night, was 33.4% in the nonoverweight, 35.8% in the overweight, and 48.2 in the obese. Among women, the corresponding figures were 37.2% in the nonoverweight, 48.3% in the overweight, and 53.6% in the obese. The authors conclude that obesity is associated with increased nocturia, more strongly among women than among men [87]. The same author and colleagues supported their initial findings stated earlier in a follow-up study. Nocturia was correlated with obesity for both sexes and with overweight for women [4]. Similar findings were reported in several other studies [8, 50, 73, 82].

Asplund assessed the relationship of nocturia to body weight in a questionnaire survey among 6,103 men and women with a mean age 73 and 72.6 years, respectively. BMI was 25.4 in men and 25.4 in women. BMI/obesity increased in parallel with increased nocturnal voiding, and both nocturnal eating and daytime loss of appetite increased correspondingly. The pattern of increase of these symptoms might support the interpretation that frequent nocturnal micturition increases the risk of obesity, partly as a consequence of its negative impact on sleep [88]. The findings of two reports from the BACH Survey showed that nocturia-related increase in prevalence with increasing BMI is in agreement with other studies [26, 46].

Interestingly, Laven and colleagues found that low subject low birth weight and abdominal adiposity (waist-to-hip ratio) are associated with increased risk of moderate to severe LUTS, including nocturia in adults [89].

Fluid Intake

Despite controversial findings, there is fair evidence of a relation between nocturia and fluid intake, particularly consumption of excess amount of fluid at evening including water, beverages, alcohol, coffee, and tea as a dietary habit. They can result in increased urinary volume, especially at night and may initiate NP that is the main cause of nocturia.

Klingler et al. found that, of 150 nocturic patients due to NP, 25.4% had high evening fluid consumption (more so in men than in women). Women had a significantly higher mean 24-h urine output than men and more women than men had a voided urine volume >2,400 ml. It is unclear whether these findings are related to different drinking habits; perhaps women tend to drink higher fluid volumes throughout the entire day, as part of what may be perceived to be a healthy lifestyle habit [7]. Mono-symptomatic polyuria >2,800 ml due to excessive fluid intake was an unexpectedly common cause nocturia in that study: in 17% of patients this was the sole etiology for nocturia. In contrast, Johnson et al. reported that nighttime fluid and coffee intake were not associated with nocturia in a sample of community-living older adults [47].

Many older people also adopt rigid drinking habits, which include fluid intake late into the night, frequently including alcohol [17]. These habits are usually associated with high nocturnal urine production and resulting nocturia [19] (Fonda 1999).

Yoshimura et al. showed that alcohol consumption impacts the prevalence of nocturia. Interestingly, moderate alcohol consumption had been reported to prevent nocturnal voiding; men drinking three times a week had a lower risk of nocturia than those drinking alcohol more, or less, often [25]. However, coffee or alcohol consumption has been shown in several recent studies not to be associated with nocturia [4, 8, 26, 47, 50, 73].

AVP is responsible for regulating urine production with a diurnal pattern in healthy people. The rhythm appears to be linked to the wake–sleep cycle rather than to the time of day. With advancing age, nocturnal secretion of AVP becomes blunted, resulting in similar day- and nighttime blood levels of AVP and hence to an increase in nighttime urine production. Also, renal concentrating capacity is reduced with age due to impaired renal tubular response to AVP. The ability of the kidney to retain sodium also decreases with advancing age: after administration of an acute water load, there is exaggerated natriuresis in older people compared with younger individuals [12].

Other hormones likely to play a role in altered renal sodium handling of elderly people are the renin–angiotensin–aldosterone system and ANP. The renin–angiotensin–aldosterone system is modulated by ANP, with high levels of ANP reducing renin secretion and leading to a decrease in plasma aldosterone [90]. It is evident that an increase in nighttime urine excretion, causing individuals to rise and void, is part of the normal aging process. Healthy people aged 62–70 years who consume a normal amount of dietary sodium have lower levels of both active plasma renin and aldosterone in the supine position than healthy individuals aged 20–30 years. The reduction in the formation of active renin in older individuals may, in part, be responsible for the decreases in the plasma concentrations of active renin and aldosterone and accompanying natriuresis during sleep-related recumbency [12].

On the other hand, the type of fluid intake appears to be important. A vasopressin-insensitive state may be caused by ethanol, resulting in a polyuric state. Caffeine-rich fluids like coffee and cola have been reported to increase smooth muscle contractility, which may aggravate existing detrusor instability and worsen frequency and nocturia [91, 38].

Smoking

The findings from several studies on relationships between nocturia and smoking are inconsistent. Asplund and Aberg reported that nocturnal micturition episodes were increased by smoking in women [92]. By contrast, Bing et al. reported that current smokers were significantly less likely to have nocturia of ≥1 voids than nonsmokers; smoking was inversely associated with nocturia in a Danish population of men and women aged 60–80 years [50]. The latter findings support results reported by Yoshimura et al. [22]. This apparent protective effect of smoking can be explained by the effect of nicotine increasing arginine vasopressin secretion that decreases nocturnal urine volume [93]. Moreover, clinical studies suggest that smoking and/or nicotine intake decreases nocturnal urine production [47, 50]. On the other hand, Tikkinen et al. reported smoking not to be associated with nocturia in the FINNO study [4]. Again, there was no relationship between nocturia and smoking in two further studies [8, 82].

Physical Activity

Until the BACH Survey [26], we had no information on a possible relationship between physical activity and nocturia, because this relationship was rejected in a prior study conducted by Schatzl and co-workers [94]. The BACH Survey demonstrated that increased physical activity was associated with decreased odds of nocturia [26]. Recently, Agarwal et al. reported that increased nighttime physical activity contributed to nondipping blood pressure patterns in chronic kidney disease (CKD) patients, possibly exacerbating nocturia [56]. However, the association between nondipping and nocturia remains unclear [18]. Interestingly, a questionnaire-based study analyzing the relationship of nocturnal micturition to regular exercise as well other factors in 3,669 women from Sweden reported lack of regular exercise to be associated with an increased number of nocturnal micturition episodes [92].

References

1. Bosch JL, Weiss JP. The prevalence and causes of nocturia. J Urol. 2010;184:440–6.
2. Van Kerrebroeck P, Abrams P, Chaikin D, Donovan J, Fonda D, Jackson S, et al. The standardisation of terminology in nocturia: report from the Standardisation Sub-committee of the International Continence Society. Neurourol Urodyn. 2002;21:179–83.
3. Van Kerrebroeck PE, Dmochowski R, FitzGerald MP, Hashim H, Norgaard JP, Robinson D, et al. Nocturia research: current status and future perspectives. Neurourol Urodyn. 2010;29(4):623–8.
4. Tikkinen KA, Auvinen A, Johnson 2nd TM, Weiss JP, Keränen T, Tiitinen A, et al. A systematic evaluation of factors associated with nocturia – the population-based FINNO study. Am J Epidemiol. 2009;170:361–8.
5. DuBeau CE, Kuchel GA, Johnson T, Palmer MH, Wagg A. Incontinence in the Frail Elderly. In: Abrams P, Cardozo L, Khoury S, Wein A, editors. Incontinence. 4th International Consultation on Incontinence. 4th ed. Plymouth: Health Publication Ltd; 2009. p. 999–1001.
6. Van Kerrebroeck P, Hashim H, Holm-Larsen T, Robinson D, Stanley N. Thinking beyond the bladder: antidiuretic treatment of nocturia. Int J Clin Pract. 2010;64:807–16.
7. Klingler HC, Heidler H, Madersbacher H, Primus G. Nocturia: an Austrian study on the multifactorial etiology of this symptom. Neurourol Urodyn. 2009;28:427–31.
8. Hsieh CH, Chen HY, Hsu CS, Chang ST, Chiang CD. Risk factors for nocturia in Taiwanese women aged 20–59 years. Taiwan J Obstet Gynecol. 2007;46:166–70.
9. Asplund R. Nocturia in relation to sleep, health, and medical treatment in the elderly. BJU Int. 2005;96 Suppl 1:15–21.
10. Hunskaar S. Epidemiology of nocturia. BJU Int. 2005;96 Suppl 1:4–7.
11. Chen FY, Dai YT, Liu CK, Yu HJ, Liu CY, Chen TH. Perception of nocturia and medical consulting behavior among community-dwelling women. Int Urogynecol J Pelvic Floor Dysfunct. 2007;18:431–6.
12. Lundgren R. Nocturia: a new perspective on an old symptom. Scand J Urol Nephrol. 2004;38:112–6.
13. Irwin DE, Milsom I, Hunskaar S, Reilly K, Kopp Z, Herschorn S, et al. Population-based survey of urinary incontinence, overactive bladder, and other lower urinary tract symptoms in five countries: results from the EPIC study. Eur Urol. 2006;50:1306–14.
14. Zhang W, Song Y, He X, Xu B, Huang H, He C, et al. Prevalence and risk factors of lower urinary tract symptoms in Fuzhou Chinese women. Eur Urol. 2005;48:309–13.
15. Asplund R, Aberg HE. Nocturia and health in women aged 40–64 years. Maturitas. 2000;35:143–8.
16. DuBeau CE, Kuchel GA, Johnson 2nd T, Palmer MH, Wagg A. Fourth International Consultation on Incontinence. Incontinence in the frail elderly: report from the 4th International Consultation on Incontinence. Neurourol Urodyn. 2010;29(1):165–78.
17. Wagg A, Andersson KE, Cardozo L, Chapple C, Kirby M, Kelleher C, et al. Nocturia: morbidity and management in adults. Int J Clin Pract. 2005;59:938–45.
18. Boongird S, Shah N, Nolin TD, Unruh ML. Nocturia and aging: diagnosis and treatment. Adv Chronic Kidney Dis. 2010;17:e27–40.
19. Fonda D. Nocturia: a disease or normal ageing? BJU Int. 1999;84 Suppl 1:13–5.
20. Tikkinen KA, Tammela TL, Huhtala H, Auvinen A. Is nocturia equally common among men and women? A population based study in Finland. J Urol. 2006;175:596–600.

21. Coyne KS, Zhou Z, Bhattacharyya SK, Thompson CL, Dhawan R, Versi E. The prevalence of nocturia and its effect on health-related quality of life and sleep in a community sample in the USA. BJU Int. 2003;92:948–54.
22. Yoshimura K, Terada N, Matsui Y, Terai A, Kinukawa N, Arai Y. Prevalence of and risk factors for nocturia: analysis of a health screening program. Int J Urol. 2004;11:282–7.
23. van Dijk L, Kooij DG, Schellevis FG. Nocturia in the Dutch adult population. BJU Int. 2002;90:644–8.
24. Homma Y, Yamaguchi T, Kondo Y, Horie S, Takahashi S, Kitamura T. Significance of nocturia in the International Prostate Symptom Score for benign prostatic hyperplasia. J Urol. 2002;167:172–6.
25. Gourova LW, van de Beek C, Spigt MG, Nieman FH, van Kerrebroeck PE. Predictive factors for nocturia in elderly men: a cross-sectional study in 21 general practices. BJU Int. 2006;97:528–32.
26. Kupelian V, Link CL, Hall SA, McKinlay JB. Are racial/ethnic disparities in the prevalence of nocturia due to socioeconomic status? Results of the BACH survey. J Urol. 2009;181:1756–63.
27. Sarma AV, Burke JP, Jacobson DJ, McGree ME, St Sauver J, Girman CJ, et al. Associations between diabetes and clinical markers of benign prostatic hyperplasia among community-dwelling Black and White men. Diabetes Care. 2008;31:476–82.
28. Platz EA, Smit E, Curhan GC, Nyberg LM, Giovannucci E. Prevalence of and racial/ethnic variation in lower urinary tract symptoms and noncancer prostate surgery in U.S. men. Urology. 2002;59(6):877–83.
29. Chuang FC, Kuo HC. Prevalence of lower urinary tract symptoms in indigenous and non-indigenous women in Eastern Taiwan. J Formos Med Assoc. 2010;109:228–36.
30. Mariappan P, Turner KJ, Sothilingam S, Rajan P, Sundram M, Stewart LH. Nocturia, nocturia indices and variables from frequency-volume charts are significantly different in Asian and Caucasian men with lower urinary tract symptoms: a prospective comparison study. BJU Int. 2007;100:332–6.
31. Massolt ET, Wooning MM, Stijnen T, Vierhout ME. Prevalence, impact on the quality of life and pathophysiological determinants of nocturia in urinary incontinent women. Int Urogynecol J Pelvic Floor Dysfunct. 2005;16:132–7.
32. Kawauchi A, Tanaka Y, Soh J, Ukimura O, Kojima M, Miki T. Causes of nocturnal urinary frequency and reasons for its increase with age in healthy older men. J Urol. 2000;163:81–4.
33. Chang SC, Lin AT, Chen KK, Chang LS. Multifactorial nature of male nocturia. Urology. 2006;67:541–4.
34. Yoong H, Sundaram M, Aida Z. Prevalence of nocturnal polyuria in patients with benign prostatis hyperplasia. Med J Malaysia. 2005;60(3):294–6.
35. Yoshimura K, Ohara H, Ichioka K, Terada N, Matsui Y, Terai A, et al. Nocturia and benign prostatic hyperplasia. Urology. 2003;61:786–90.
36. Djavan B, Fong YK, Chaudry A, Reissigl A, Anagnostou T, Bagheri F, et al. Progression delay in men with mild symptoms of bladder outlet obstruction: a comparative study of phytotherapy and watchful waiting. World J Urol. 2005;23:253–6.
37. Johnson TM, Jones K, Williford WO, Kutner MH, Issa MM, Lepor H. Changes in nocturia from medical treatment of benign prostatic hyperplasia: secondary analysis of the Department of Veterans Affairs Cooperative Study Trial. J Urol. 2003;170:145–8.
38. Hvistendahl GM, Djurhuus JC. Female nocturia. Int Urol Nephrol. 2002;33:179–86.
39. Weiss JP, Blaivas JG, Stember DS, Brooks MM. Nocturia in adults: etiology and classification. Neurourol Urodyn. 1998;17:467–72.
40. Brubaker L, FitzGerald MP. Nocturnal polyuria and nocturia relief in patients treated with solifenacin for overactive bladder symptoms. Int Urogynecol J Pelvic Floor Dysfunct. 2007;18:737–41.
41. Eckford SD, Carter PG, Jackson SR, Penney MD, Abrams P. An open, in-patient incremental safety and efficacy study of desmopressin in women with multiple sclerosis and nocturia. Br J Urol. 1995;76(4):459–63.

42. Resnick NM, Yalla SV. Detrusor hyperactivity with impaired contractile function. An unrecognized but common cause of incontinence in elderly patients. JAMA. 1987;257:3076–81.
43. Stember DS, Weiss JP, Lee CL, Blaivas JG. Nocturia in men. Int J Clin Pract Suppl. 2007;155:17–22.
44. Reynard JM, Cannon A, Yang Q, Abrams P. A novel therapy for nocturnal polyuria: a double-blind randomized trial of frusemide against placebo. Br J Urol. 1998;81:215–8.
45. Rembratt A, Norgaard JP, Andersson KE. Nocturia and associated morbidity in a community-dwelling elderly population. BJU Int. 2003;92:726–30.
46. Fitzgerald MP, Litman HJ, Link CL, et al. The association of nocturia with cardiac disease, diabetes, body mass index, age and diuretic use: results from the BACH survey. J Urol. 2007;177:1385–9.
47. Johnson TM, Sattin RW, Pamelee P, Fultz NH, Ouslander JG. Evaluating potentially modifiable risk factors for prevalent and incident nocturia in older adults. J Am Geriatr Soc. 2005;53:1011–116.
48. Rembratt A, Norgaard JP, Andersson KE. Differences between nocturics and non-nocturics in voiding patterns: an analysis of frequency-volume charts from community-dwelling elderly. BJU Int. 2003;91:45–50.
49. Blanker MH, Bohnen AM, Groeneveld FP, Bernsen RM, Prins A, Ruud Bosch JL. Normal voiding patterns and determinants of increased diurnal and nocturnal voiding frequency in elderly men. J Urol. 2000;164:1201–5.
50. Bing MH, Moller LA, Jennum P, Mortensen S, Lose G. Nocturia and associated morbidity in a Danish population of men and women aged 60–80 years. BJU Int. 2008;102:808–14.
51. Asplund R. Nocturia, nocturnal polyuria, and sleep quality in the elderly. J Psychosom Res. 2004;56:517–25.
52. Fujikawa K, Kasahara M, Matsui Y, Takeuchi H. Human atrial natriureticpeptide is a useful criterion in treatment of nocturia. Scand J Urol Nephrol. 2001;35:310–3.
53. Torimoto K, Hirayama A, Samma S, Yoshida K, Fujimoto K, Hirao Y. The relationship between nocturnal polyuria and the distribution of body fluid: assessment by bioelectric impedance analysis. J Urol. 2009;181:219–24.
54. Ali A, Snape J. Nocturia in older people: a review of causes, consequences, assessment and management. Int J Clin Pract. 2004;58:366–73.
55. McKeigue PM, Reynard JM. Relation of nocturnal polyuria of the elderly to essential hypertension. Lancet. 2000;355:486–8.
56. Agarwal R, Light RP, Bills JE, Hummel LA. Nocturia, nocturnal activity, and nondipping. Hyprtension. 2009;54:646–51.
57. McNicholas WT, Bonsigore MR. Management Committee of EU COST ACTION B26. Sleep apnoea as an independent risk factor for cardiovascular disease: current evidence, basic mechanisms and research priorities. Eur Respir J. 2007;29:156–78.
58. Asplund R. Mortality in the elderly in relation to nocturnal micturition. BJU Int. 1999;84:297–301.
59. Bursztyn M, Jacob J, Stessman J. Usefulness of nocturia as a mortality risk factor for coronary heart disease among persons born in 1920 or 1921. Am J Cardiol. 2006;98:1311–5.
60. Weiss JP, Blaivas JG. Nocturia. J Urol. 2000;163:5–12.
61. Tikkinen KA, Johnson 2nd TM, Tammela TL, Sintonen H, Haukka J, Huhtala H, et al. Nocturia frequency, bother, and quality of life: how often is too often? A population-based study in Finland. Eur Urol. 2010;57:488–96.
62. Oztura I, Kaynak D, Kaynak HC. Nocturia in sleep-disordered breathing. Sleep Med. 2006;7:362–7.
63. Hajduk IA, Strollo Jr PJ, Jasani RR, Atwood Jr CW, Houck PR, Sanders MH. Prevalence and predictors of nocturia in obstructive sleep apnea-hypopnea syndrome–a retrospective study. Sleep. 2003;26:61–4.
64. Robinson D. Nocturia in women. Int J Clin Pract Suppl. 2007;155:23–31.
65. Pressman MR, Figueroa WG, Kendrick-Mohamed J, Greenspon LW, Peterson DD. Nocturia. A rarely recognized symptom of sleep apnea and other occult sleep disorders. Arch Intern Med. 1996;156(5):545–50.

66. Lowenstein L, Kenton K, Brubaker L, Pillar G, Undevia N, Mueller ER, et al. The relationship between obstructive sleep apnea, nocturia, and daytime overactive bladder syndrome in women. Am J Obstet Gynecol. 2008;198:598.e1–5.
67. Umlauf MG, Chasens ER, Greevy RA, Arnold J, Burgio KL, Pillion DJ. Obstructive sleep apnea, nocturia and polyuria in older adults. Sleep. 2004;27:139–44.
68. Moriyama Y, Miwa K, Tanaka H, Fujihiro S, Nishino Y, Deguchi T. Nocturia in men less than 50 years of age may be associated with obstructive sleep apnea syndrome. Urology. 2008;71:1096–8.
69. Bliwise DL, Foley DJ, Vitiello MV, Ansari FP, Ancoli-Israel S, Walsh JK. Nocturia and disturbed sleep in the elderly. Sleep Med. 2009;10(5):540–8.
70. Yoshimura K, Oka Y, Kamoto T, Yoshimura K, Ogawa O. Differences and associations between nocturnal voiding/nocturia and sleep disorders. BJU Int. 2010;106:232–7.
71. Kinn AC, Harlid R. Snoring as a cause of nocturia in men with lower urinary tract symptoms. Eur Urol. 2003;43:696–701.
72. Gopal M, Sammel MD, Pien G, Gracia C, Freeman EW, Lin H, et al. Investigating the associations between nocturia and sleep disorders in perimenopausal women. J Urol. 2008;180:2063–7.
73. Burgio KL, Johnson 2nd TM, Goode PS, Markland AD, Richter HE, Roth DL, et al. Prevalence and correlates of nocturia in community-dwelling older adults. J Am Geriatr Soc. 2010;58:861–6.
74. Umlauf M, Kurtzer E, Valappil T, Burgio K, Pillion D, Goode P. Sleep-disordered breathing as a mechanism for nocturia: preliminary findings. Ostomy Wound Manage. 1999;45:52–60.
75. Margel D, Lifshitz D, Brown N, Lask D, Livne PM, Tal R. Predictors of nocturia quality of life before and shortly after prostatectomy. Urology. 2007;70:493–7.
76. Chen CY, Hsu CC, Pei YC, Yu CC, Chen YS, Chen CL. Nocturia is an independent predictor of severe obstructive sleep apnea in patients with ischemic stroke. J Neurol. 2010;258(2):189–94. doi:10.1007/s00415-010-5705-2.
77. Hardin-Fanning F, Gross JC. The effects of sleep-disordered breathing symptoms on voiding patterns in stroke patients. Urol Nurs. 2007;27:221–4.
78. Koseoglu H, Aslan G, Ozdemir I, Esen A. Nocturnal polyuria in patients with lower urinary tract symptoms and response to alpha-blocker therapy. Urology. 2006;67:1188–92.
79. Marinkovic SP, Gillen LM, Stanton SL. Managing nocturia. BMJ. 2004;328:1063–6.
80. Petros P. The female pelvic floor; function, dysfunction and management according to the integral theory. 2nd ed. Heidelberg, Germany: Springer Medizin Verlag; 2007.
81. Tikkinen KA, Auvinen A, Tiitinen A, Valpas A, Johnson 2nd TM, Tammela TL. Reproductive factors associated with nocturia and urinary urgency in women – a population-based study in Finland. Am J Obstet Gynecol. 2008;199:153.e1–153.e12 [electronic article].
82. Shiri R, Hakama M, Häkkinen J, Auvinen A, Huhtala H, Tammela TL, et al. The effects of lifestyle factors on the incidence of nocturia. J Urol. 2008;180:2059–62.
83. Soda T, Masui K, Okuno H, Terai A, Ogawa O, Yoshimura K. Efficacy of nondrug lifestyle measures for the treatment of nocturia. J Urol. 2010;184:1000–4.
84. Nakagawa H, Niu K, Hozawa A, Ikeda Y, Kaiho Y, Ohmori-Matsuda K, et al. Impact of nocturia on bone fracture and mortality in older individuals: a Japanese longitudinal cohort study. J Urol. 2010;184:1413–8.
85. Nakagawa H, Niu K, Hozawa A, Ikeda Y, Kaiho Y, Masuda-Ohmori K, et al. Association between nocturia and mortality in a community-dwelling elderly population aged 70 years and over: results of a 3-year prospective cohort study in Japan. J Urol. 2009;181:8.
86. Ashok K, Wang A. Nocturia. Obstet Gynecol Surv. 2010;65:403–7.
87. Tikkinen KA, Auvinen A, Huhtala H, Tammela TL. Nocturia and obesity: a population-based study in Finland. Am J Epidemiol. 2006;163:1003–11.
88. Asplund R. Obesity in elderly people with nocturia: cause or consequence? Can J Urol. 2007;14:3424–8.
89. Laven BA, Orsini N, Andersson SO, Johansson JE, Gerber GS, Wolk A. Birth weight, abdominal obesity and the risk of lower urinary tract symptoms in a population based study of Swedish men. J Urol. 2008;179:1891–5.
90. Rubattu S, Volpe M. The atrial natriuretic peptide: a changing view. J Hypertens. 2001;19:1923–31.

91. Arya LA, Myers DL, Jackson ND. Dietary caffeine intake and the risk for detrusor instability: a case-control study. Obstet Gynecol. 2000;96:85–9.
92. Asplund R, Aberg HE. Nocturia in relation to body mass index, smoking and some other lifestyle factors in women. Climacteric. 2004;7:267–73.
93. Fuxe K, Andersson K, Eneroth P, Harfstrand A, Agnati LF. Neuroendocrine actions of nicotine and of exposure to cigarette smoke: medical implications. Psychoneuroendocrinology. 1989;14:19–41.
94. Schatzl G, Temml C, Schmidbauer J, Dolezal B, Haidinger G, Madersbacher S. Cross-sectional study of nocturia in both sexes: analysis of a voluntary health screening project. Urology. 2000;56:71–5.

Chapter 3
Nocturia and Sleep Disorders: Morbidity, Mortality, Quality of Life and Economics

Sonia Ancoli-Israel, Donald L. Bliwise, and Jens Peter Nørgaard

Keywords Sleep • Sleep disorders • Nocturia • Sleep apnea • Morbidity • Mortality • Sleep duration • Sleep efficiency • Falls and fractures

Introduction

Nocturia has been associated with poor daytime function, decreased quality of life, and mortality. Nocturia is also known to disrupt sleep and poor sleep is also associated with these same consequences. The relationship between nocturia and sleep, the consequences of each, and the relevance of sleep disorders for patients with nocturia present complex problems for analysis. This chapter will seek to explore the many issues relating to the clinical impact of nocturia and the role that sleep plays in these issues.

Morbidity and Mortality in Nocturia

Studies have consistently reported that nocturia is associated with an elevated risk of mortality. This is not surprising since nocturia can be a symptom of several serious illnesses, including heart disease, kidney disease, diabetes mellitus, and hypertension

---

S. Ancoli-Israel, PhD (✉)
Department of Psychiatry, University of California, San Diego, 9500 Gilman Drive,
La Jolla, CA 92093-0733, USA
e-mail: sancoliisrael@ucsd.edu

D.L. Bliwise, PhD
Psychiatry/Behavioral Sciences, and Nursing; Director, Program in Sleep, Aging and Chronobiology, Emory University School of Medicine, Wesley Woods Health Center, 1841 Clifton Road, Room 509, Atlanta, Georgia 30329, USA

J.P. Nørgaard, MD, DMSc
Medical Sciences Urology, Ferring International Pharmascience Center, Copenhagen, Denmark

[1]. However, a number of studies have now demonstrated an association between nocturia and mortality even when controlling for several key comorbidities.

In one of the first such studies [2], Asplund found that amongst elderly Swedes, those with nocturia ≥3 voids per night were at increased risk of death over a 54-month period, and that this association was independent of age, general health, changes in health during the 5 years before the survey, cardiac diseases, stroke, and diabetes. Other similar studies have corroborated these findings. Nakagawa and colleagues [3], for example, found that ≥2 voids per night were associated with increased mortality risk in an elderly Japanese community-based sample, despite analyses adjusted for age, gender, body mass index (BMI), diabetes, smoking status, coronary disease, renal disease, stroke, and use of tranquilizers, hypnotics and diuretics (hazard ratio [HR] 1.98; 95% confidence interval [CI] 1.09–3.59; $p=0.03$). Further studies have demonstrated a relationship between nocturia and mortality in specific patient populations. For instance, in a cohort of 70-year olds with coronary heart disease, nocturia predicted a doubled mortality rate over 12 years (10% lower survival rate for those with nocturia vs. those without), controlling for known mortality risk factors such as diabetes mellitus and heart failure [4].

As detailed above, most studies to date have focused on the relationship between nocturia and mortality rates amongst the elderly. However, a recent study using data from the Third National Health and Nutrition Examination Survey (NHANES III) investigated nocturia in relation to mortality rates across the full adult age range of the U.S. civilian population (≥20 years old) [5]. The novel finding in this study was that nocturia was not just a strong independent predictor of mortality (adjusting for BMI, cardiovascular disease, diabetes, hypertension, and prescription medications), but that this association was at its strongest in younger men and women (<65 years). Mortality risk also increased with increased number of voids per night.

Therefore, mounting evidence suggests that nocturia in both the elderly and also in younger adults is a predictor of mortality and may be a marker of poor overall health. Clearly, no study has yet performed analyses so thorough that they have controlled for all possible confounding comorbidities which might compromise the independence of the association between nocturia and mortality. However, most of the major factors which might be suspected to mediate the relationship have in fact been found not to explain the link.

The question remains then as to what can explain the observation that those with two or more voids per night are at increased risk of poor health and reduced survival independent of comorbid disease. One possibility is that sleep, which is a key factor both in nocturia and in health, may mediate this relationship.

Nocturia, Functioning, and Quality of Life

A frequently reported and acknowledged observation is that people with nocturia have significantly reduced levels of daytime functioning and quality of life (QoL) [6].

In a community study of 663 Taiwanese adults with nocturia [7], QoL decreased with increasing episodes of nocturia. Importantly, the impact of nocturia on QoL was greatest for those experiencing at least two episodes per night. These findings

Table 3.1 Age-standardized proportions for degree of bother by frequency of nocturia in both sexes [9]

Voids per night (%)	Degree of bother from nocturia			
	None	Small	Moderate	Major
1	52.2	41.1	5.9	0.7
2	29.3	53.8	13.9	3.1
3	17.4	26.7	41.9	14.0
≥4	11.3	7.0	46.0	35.7

Age standardization was performed using the age structure of Finland at the beginning of 2004

Reprinted from Eur Urol, 57/3, Tikkinen KAO et al., Nocturia frequency, bother and quality of life: how often is too often? A population-based study in Finland, 488–496. Copyright 2010, with permission from Elsevier

were consistent with a U.S. study of 1,214 women [8], which showed that nocturia had a significant impact in patients with at least two night-time voids. A Finnish study of nearly 3,500 adults found that bother was reported by the majority of respondents experiencing ≥2 voids per night (Table 3.1), again confirming that this level of severity is of clinical relevance [9].

These data all suggest that irrespective of gender or geographical background, nocturia adversely affects QoL. Furthermore, the causal relationship between nocturia, sleep disturbance, and reduced QoL is demonstrated by the observation that the extent of sleep disturbance caused by nocturia is an independent predictor of lower QoL [7].

Sleep: The Missing Link?

The direct link between poor sleep and fatigue, with implications for alertness and QoL, is widely acknowledged. It is likely, therefore, that the effects of nocturia on QoL might be mediated by poor sleep.

Disruptions to sleep can take many forms and include changes in sleep duration, the number of awakenings during sleep, and sleep efficiency (the proportion of time in bed that is spent asleep). Many types of research converge to indicate the importance of such sleep parameters for a person's functioning and overall health. However, a weakness of many of the traditional epidemiological studies of sleep problems was that the issue of nocturia was largely ignored, despite it being the most widely reported cause of sleep disturbance on a nightly or almost nightly basis [10].

Quantity of Sleep: Sleep Duration

Short sleep duration has been found to be associated with abnormalities of glucose metabolism and endocrine function [11]. A mean sleep duration of less than 6 h, as well as a long duration of sleep over 9 h, was linked with a significantly raised prevalence of impaired glucose tolerance and type 2 diabetes mellitus in a sample of 1,486 adults over 53 years (a U-shaped relationship; Fig. 3.1) [12]. This association remained even after adjustment for various potential confounders such as age, waist

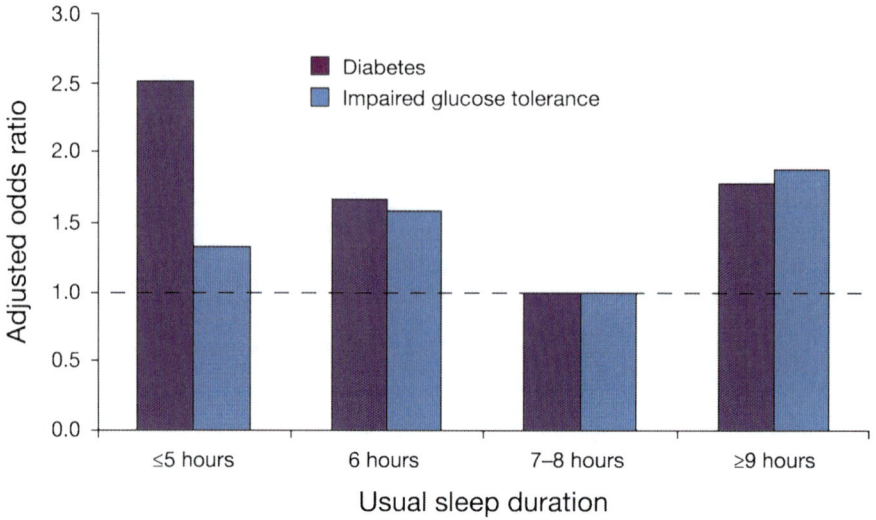

Fig. 3.1 Short and long sleep duration are associated with diabetes mellitus and impaired glucose tolerance [12]. Odds ratio adjusted for age, age [2], sex, race/ethnicity, apnea/hypopnea index, study site, and waist girth. Reprinted by permission from

girth, systolic blood pressure, coronary heart disease, heart failure or stroke, caffeine and alcohol consumption, depression, and nocturia. It has been replicated in several studies with both subjective and objective measures of sleep duration [13–17], and in a recent meta-analysis of prospective studies of sleep disturbance and incidence of type 2 diabetes [18].

Similar findings regarding short sleep duration are reported in relation to obesity [19] and hypertension [20, 21]. Blood pressure falls when sleep begins and remains 10–20% below normal waking levels until rising quickly with awakening [22, 23].

One hypothesis as to the mechanism of the link between reduced sleep duration and these poor metabolic and endocrine health outcomes arises from experimental studies showing that sleep deprivation decreases leptin, increases ghrelin, increases appetite, attenuates insulin sensitivity, and increases blood pressure [22].

Obesity, diabetes, and cardiovascular disease are characterized to some extent by inflammatory processes. Experimental sleep deprivation has also been shown to lead to increased peripheral circulation of leukocytes and interleukin, suggesting that reduced sleep duration may cause low-grade inflammation. Acute and short-term partial sleep deprivation also resulted in elevated C-reactive protein (a marker of acute-phase response to inflammation) [24, 25]. This may have an impact upon cardiovascular disease and other conditions including cancer. Recent reports indicate that disease resistance may have played a major role in the evolution of mammalian sleep. It has been suggested that "sleep fuels the immune system," since there is a strong association between the daily sleep time of a species and both an increased white blood cell count and reduced infection status [26]. As a logical correlate of these associations between sleep duration and morbidity, a U-shaped relationship with mortality has also been found (see Fig. 3.2) [27, 28]. A large body of

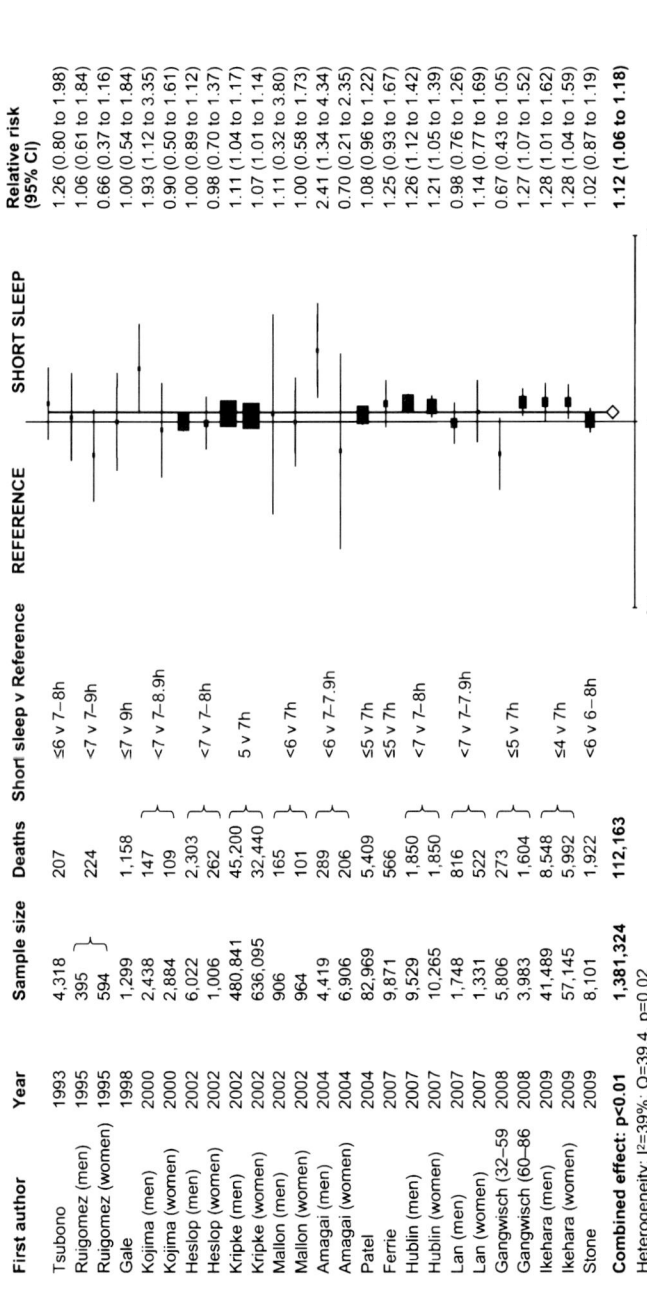

Fig. 3.2 Forest plot showing the risk of death associated with short duration of sleep compared with the reference group in 25 population cohorts from 15 published prospective studies including 1,381,324 participants and 112,163 events. Results are expressed as relative risk (RR) and 95% confidence intervals (CI). The RR and CI of the individual studies are depicted relative to the *vertical line* representing an RR of 1 (i.e., no difference in risk). The *vertical line* represented by *diamond* shows the RR of the pooled analysis. This indicates that even though several individual studies find a reduced risk of death, the pooled analysis (which takes into consideration the sample size/statistical power of the studies) documents an increased risk of death. Cappuccio FP et al. Sleep duration and all-cause mortality: a systematic review and meta-analysis of prospective studies. Sleep 33(5):585–592. Copyright 2010 Reproduced with permission of American Academy of Sleep Medicine via Copyright Clearance Center

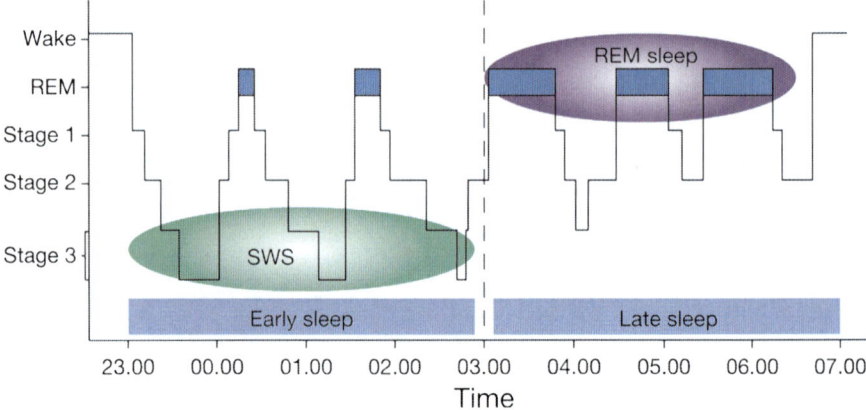

Fig. 3.3 Sleep stages, including slow-wave sleep [36]. Adapted from Diekelmann and Born 2010 [36]. Reprinted by permission from Macmillan Publishers Ltd: Diekelmann S and Born J. The memory function of sleep. Nat Rev Neurosci 11(2):114–126, copyright 2010

evidence suggests that the relationship between short sleep duration and mortality may result from the detrimental physiological impact of inadequate sleep.

Sleep Duration in Nocturia

Reports indicate that there is a significant reduction in sleep duration with increasing nocturia severity [29, 30]. However, few studies compare sleep duration in people with nocturia versus controls. It has been suggested that overall length of sleep may in fact be similar or even increased in those with nocturia, especially in retired elderly, as they may sleep longer in the morning to compensate for the increased awakenings during the night. Sleep duration is, therefore, perhaps not the most reliable parameter by which to assess sleep quality in nocturia since it may be insensitive to the presence of sleep problems relating to the interruption of the sleep period.

Normal Sleep Architecture

The sleep period has a characteristic "architecture" incorporating various stages and types of sleep. More than 50 years ago, Aserinsky and Kleitman documented the existence of two distinct sleep states, which were termed rapid eye movement (REM) and nonrapid eye movement (NREM) [31]. According to the American Academy of Sleep Medicine's 2007 standards, NREM, which constitutes 75% of total sleep time, is further subdivided into three states representing progression from light to deeper sleep: stage N1, transition from wakefulness to sleep; stage N2, light sleep; and stage N3, deep sleep or slow wave sleep (SWS; Fig. 3.3). REM and NREM alternate over a period of four to six cycles during a typical night's sleep, with SWS predominating in the first 3–4 h of the night and REM sleep predominating in the last third of the night [32–34]. Although the true function of each stage of sleep is not known, SWS or REM sleep deprivation on one night leads to a compensatory rebound the following night, suggesting that these stages of sleep are important. SWS is thought to be related to restorative sleep and REM sleep is believed to be related to memory consolidation [35].

Measures of Sleep

Sleep duration: SWS can only be measured with electroencephalographic assessment. Since most SWS occurs during the first 4 h of the night, waking up to void in the beginning of the sleep period may result in disrupted sleep patterns and reduced SWS, although the possibility exists that SWS interruption in the first portion of the night by nocturia may be compensated by SWS rebound during the second portion of the night.

Sleep efficiency: A related but distinct sleep parameter is sleep efficiency. This is calculated as the proportion of time spent in bed that is spent asleep, and therefore may give a better indication of sleep problems than total sleep duration. To illustrate this with an example, if a man spends 9 h in bed every night, achieving four bouts of sleep totaling 7 h (e.g., three 2-h periods and one 1-h period), his total sleep duration is considered normal, whereas his sleep efficiency of 78% is suboptimal. Sleep efficiency therefore has greater sensitivity to abnormalities in sleep patterns, including interrupted sleep. More information, however, would be required to specify what a sleep efficiency of 78% denotes – for example, another man who takes 2 h to fall to sleep, then sleeps for 7 h before rising, would have the same sleep efficiency, but an entirely different sleep pattern predominated by a difficulty initiating sleep (and increased sleep latency) rather than a lack of sleep continuity.

The importance of considering as many sleep parameters as possible is therefore clear, since all have their limitations as an accurate and comprehensive reflection of sleep quality. However, they all give us valuable information, and the importance of SWS and sleep efficiency for daytime performance and for health has been demonstrated by numerous studies.

SWS: Several reports have indicated a link between SWS, learning, and memory consolidation [36–39]. A recent study also demonstrated that SWS preceding a task prospectively facilitates the encoding of new information by the hippocampus. It is possible, though, that some of the effects reported are due to changes in sleep continuity rather than SWS specifically, but the influence of each of these parameters as distinct from the other is difficult to discern [40]. Nevertheless, a negative effect of sleep interruption, rather than simply sleep duration, is consistently reported. Furthermore, waking during SWS has been linked with attenuation of prepulse inhibition of the startle reflex (prepulse inhibition is the phenomenon whereby a weaker prestimulus inhibits the startle reaction to a subsequent stronger stimulus), [30] and disruption of SWS is associated with fatigue and discomfort irrespective of a reduction in total sleep time [41].

Indeed, SWS seems to be of great relevance to health in general. For example, animal models indicate that there is an elevation in levels of SWS during infection

[42], suggesting that the SWS phase is important for immunity and disease resistance. Toth also found that a failure to exhibit increases in SWS during infection with *Escherichia-coli*, *Streptomyces aureus*, or *Candida albicans* correlated with increased rates of mortality in rabbits [43]. In humans, SWS is increased across the night by very low, subpyrogenic doses of endotoxin (less than one-thousandth of the per-bodyweight dose elicits sleep responses in rats) [44]. As the dose of endotoxin increases there are transient increases in SWS, lasting around 1 h [45, 46].

The importance of SWS has also been highlighted in other areas. Just as studies of sleep duration indicate a link with metabolic outcomes, studies of SWS interruption implicate this sleep phase in the risk of type 2 diabetes due to an apparent involvement of SWS in glucose homeostasis [11, 47, 48]. In young healthy adults, disruption of SWS for a period of three nights without alterations to total sleep quantity was associated with a reduction in glucose clearance, which was not compensated for by an increase in insulin secretion. Moreover, the magnitude of the reduction in SWS correlated with the extent of the reduction in insulin sensitivity (Fig. 3.4). These findings support a relationship between SWS reduction and the risk for type 2 diabetes.

SWS is also important for blood pressure and nocturnal dipping of blood pressure. In one study, mean arterial dipping was attenuated during the first half of the sleep period after experimental SWS deprivation ($p<0.05$) [49]. The authors conclude that in healthy humans, the magnitude of nocturnal blood pressure dipping is significantly affected by sleep depth.

Impaired sleep efficiency is associated with cognitive impairment in older women [50] and poorer physical function in older men [51]. Consistent with the apparent effects of reduced sleep duration and reduced SWS, reduced sleep efficiency has also been found to be associated with reduced immunity. For example, Cohen et al. [52] investigated 153 participants who were administered nasal drops containing a rhinovirus, quarantined and monitored on the day before and for 5 days following exposure for development of a clinical cold (infection in the presence of objective signs of illness). As well as finding a relationship between susceptibility and reduced sleep duration, those with sleep efficiency of <92% were 5.50 times (95% CI: 2.08–14.48) more likely to develop a cold than those with efficiencies ≥98%.

As with sleep duration and reduced SWS, difficulty maintaining sleep (which would therefore lead to a reduced sleep efficiency) is also associated with increased risk for type 2 diabetes (Fig. 3.5) [18]. All such findings linking nocturnal awakenings with poor health are in line with results from a telephone survey in the United States, in which awakenings were associated with significantly more days of sick leave (waking every night: 37.4 days; 5–6 nights per week: 36.4; 3–4 nights per week: 33.3) compared with awakening fewer than 3 days per week (26.6, $p<0.001$) [53]. This is echoed by the observation that women aged 40–64 years in Sweden who void ≥3 times per night visit a doctor twice as often as those without nocturia, and take sick leave for 75 versus 15 days per year [54].

Furthermore, healthy older adults with sleep efficiency <80% are at 1.93 times greater mortality risk than those with efficiency ≥80%, which is significant even when controlling for factors such as baseline medical burden, age, and gender ($p=0.014$, CI 1.14–3.25; Fig. 3.6) [55].

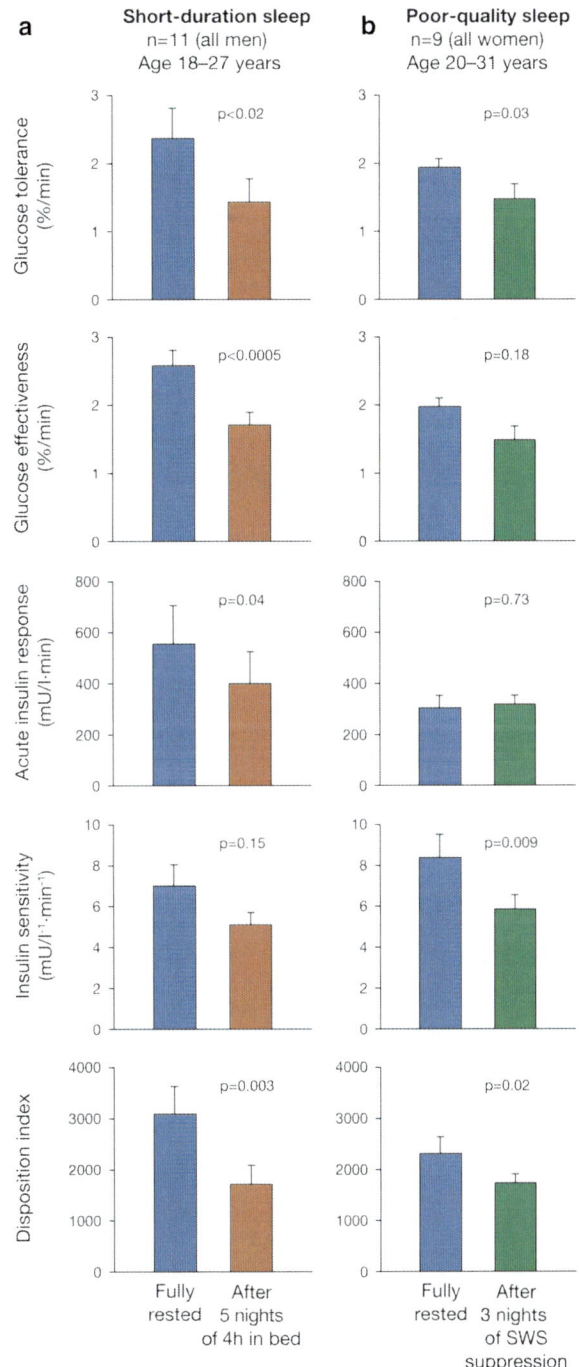

Fig. 3.4 Results from intravenous glucose tolerance tests in healthy individuals [48] when fully rested and after manipulation of sleep duration (**a**) [11] or sleep quality via SWS (**b**) [47]. SWS, slow-wave sleep. (**a**) Reprinted by permission from Macmillan Publishers Ltd: Spiegel K et al. Effects of poor and short sleep on glucose metabolism and obesity risk. Nat Rev Endocrinol 5(5):253–261, copyright 2009. (**b**) Tasali E et al. Slow-wave sleep and the risk of type 2 diabetes in humans. Proc Natl Acad Sci 105:1044–1049. Copyright 2008 National Academy of Sciences, USA

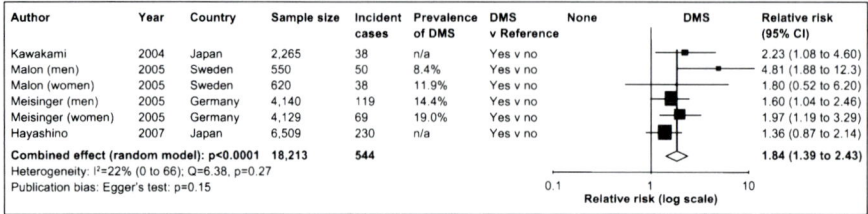

Fig. 3.5 Difficulty in maintaining sleep and increased incidence of type 2 diabetes [18]. Forest plot showing the risk of type 2 diabetes associated with difficulty maintaining sleep (DMS) compared with no difficulty (reference group) in six population cohorts from four published studies. Results are expressed as relative risk (RR) and 95% confidence intervals (CI). Copyright 2010 American Diabetes Association. From Diabetes Care, Vol. 33, 2010; 414–420. Reproduced by permission of The American Diabetes Association

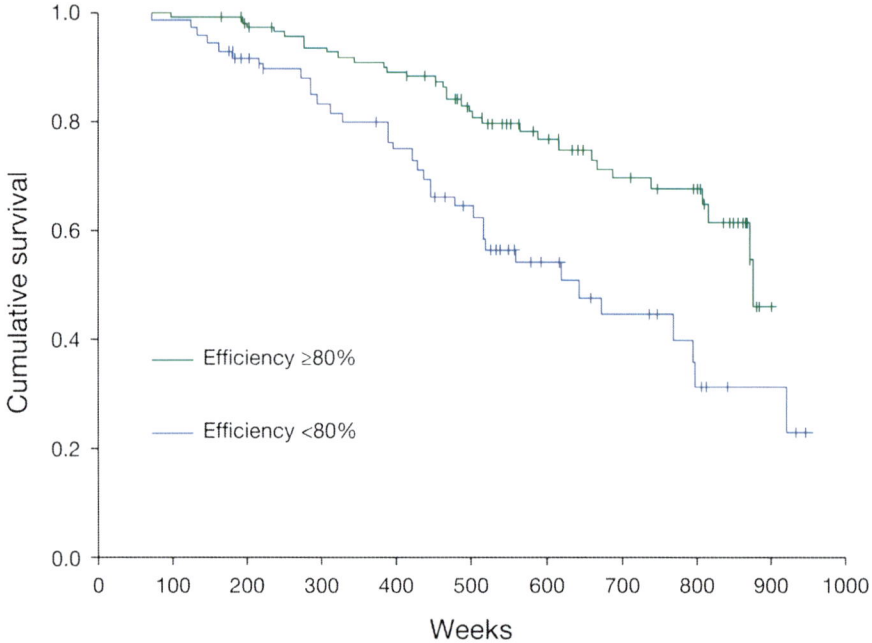

Fig. 3.6 Survival as a function of sleep efficiency [55]. Mean survival times were 624 weeks and 754 weeks for lesser and greater sleep efficiency, respectively. + = censored observation. Dew MA et al. Healthy older adults' sleep predicts all-cause mortality at 4 to 19 years of follow-up. Psychosom Med 2003;65(1):63–73. Reprinted with permission from Wolters Kluwer Health

Sleep Continuity in Nocturia

While there are only a limited number of studies looking specifically at sleep continuity and related sleep parameters in nocturia, the condition inevitably fragments sleep repeatedly during the night, and it is reported to be the most frequent reason for nocturnal awakenings in adults [10, 53, 56]. On average, people with ≥2 voids per

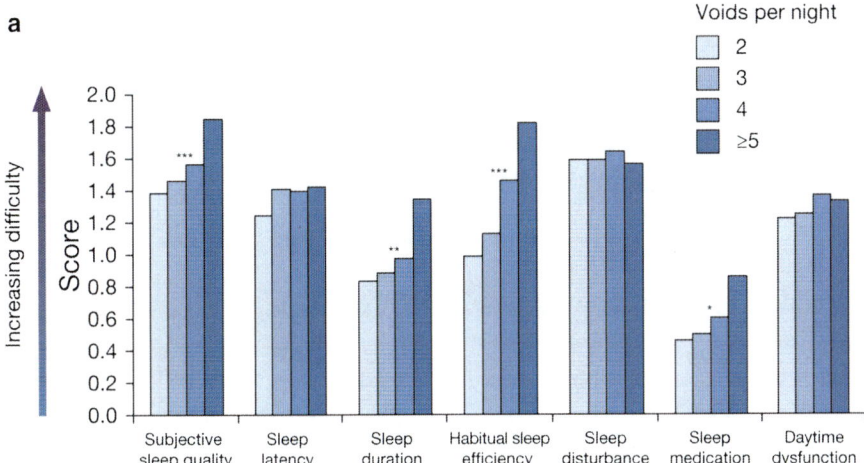

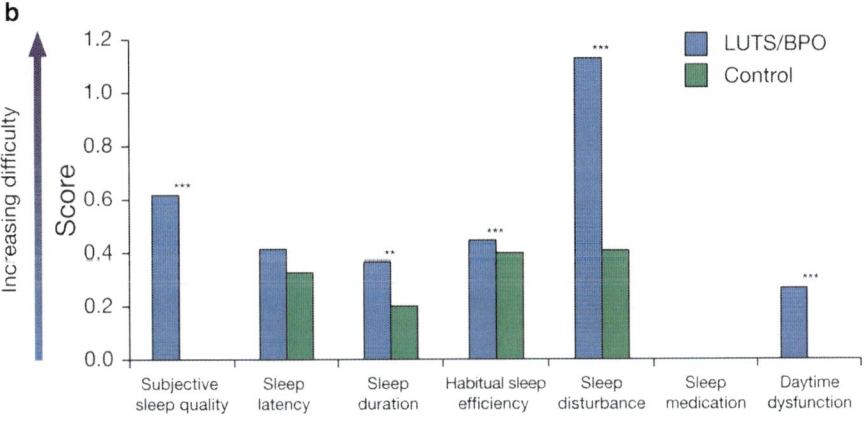

Fig. 3.7 Pittsburgh Sleep Quality Index (PSQI) scores in two studies of adults with nocturia [29, 30]. Figures show PSQI domain scores (**a**) with increasing nocturia severity in men and women ($n = 776$) [29] and (**b**) for men with nocturia (≥ 2 episodes per night; $n = 61$) compared with controls with no nocturia ($n = 48$) [30]. PSQI domain score range: 0 (no difficulty) to 3 (severe difficulty). Scores are standardized versions of areas routinely assessed during clinical interviews of patients with sleep/wake complaints. (**a**) Ancoli-Israel S et al. Does the use of sleep questionnaires add to our knowledge about the impact of nocturia? Neurourol Urodyn 2009;28(7): 635–636. Reprinted with permission from John Wiley & Sons, Inc

night recruited to nocturia trials report waking for the first void after around 2.5 h of sleep [57]. This means that it is likely that SWS, which predominates in the early part of the night, is often interrupted, although studies directly assessing SWS in these patients are lacking. However, subjectively reported sleep efficiency has been shown to decline significantly with increasing nocturia severity ($p < 0.0001$), along with several other measures of sleep quality (Fig. 3.7) [29]. Cai et al. [30] also reported that men with nocturia of ≥2 voids per night had significantly reduced sleep efficiency compared with controls, as well as significant impairments in most other sleep subscales (including sleep quality, duration, disturbance, and daytime dysfunction; Fig. 3.7). Similarly, in a separate sample of men with nocturia and benign prostatic hyperplasia, the sleep efficiency index decreased with nocturia frequency ($89.8 \pm 11.3\%$ for two nocturia episodes vs. $80.4 \pm 17.3\%$ for five nocturia episodes or more, $p<0.001$) [58].

Falls and Fractures

Poor sleep is associated with increased risk of falls in the elderly [59]. There is also an increased likelihood of falls among older people with nocturia, which may arise directly from the necessity to make trips to the bathroom at night and/or sleepiness during the day as a result of disrupted sleep. A cross-sectional study of 988 women and 520 men showed that having at least two or three voids per night approximately doubled the risk of falls (at least two voids: odds ratio [OR] 1.84, 95% CI 1.05, 3.22; at least three voids: OR 2.15, 95% CI 1.04, 4.44) [60]. Studies have shown a significant positive association between the frequency of voiding each night and the prevalence of bone fractures [3, 61, 62], with two voids or more per night associated with a greater than twofold increase in the risk of fractures (HR 2.01 [95% CI 1.04–3.87]) and fall-related fractures (HR 2.20 [95% CI 1.04–4.68]) in one study [3]. Another recent study also found the increased risk of hip fractures in men with nocturia to be age-independent [63]. In turn, hip fractures have been reported to be associated with an in-hospital mortality rate of 5.3% [64], demonstrating that such injuries can have serious implications and are sometimes fatal. Other kinds of accidents and injuries, such as traffic and workplace accidents, are also more common when sleep is impaired [65]. Fatigue is estimated to be involved in 16–60% of road accidents, and driving after moderate sleep deprivation is reported to be at least as dangerous as low-level alcohol intoxication [66]. As such, the effects of nocturia on sleep may have serious consequences not only in terms of falls, but also other types of injury due to reduced alertness.

Sleep Apnea

The relationship between sleep and nocturia is bidirectional. Not only does nocturnal voiding cause sleep problems including comorbid insomnia, primary sleep disorders can in fact cause nocturia. A key example of this is sleep apnea. Sleep apnea is a condition where breathing ceases entirely or is otherwise diminished during sleep. Each breathing event typically lasts 10–20 s or more, and these pauses can occur 20 to 30 times or more an hour. The most frequent type of sleep apnea is obstructive sleep apnea (OSA), where the throat muscles collapse, leading to interruptions in breathing which may cause a drop in blood oxygen levels [67].

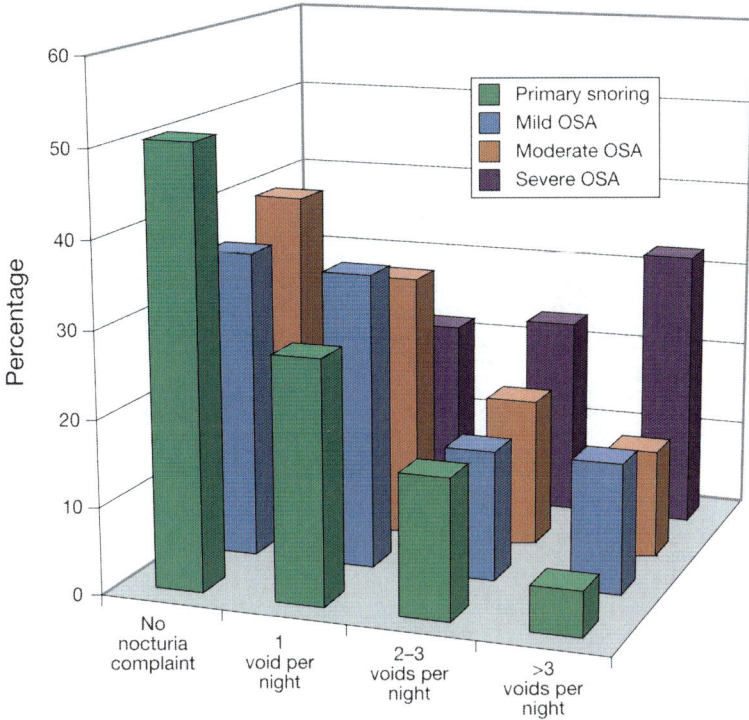

Fig. 3.8 Frequency of nocturnal voiding according to OSA syndrome severity [68]. Nocturia of more than three episodes per night was significantly more reported by severe obstructive sleep apnea (OSA) patients than other groups of OSA patients ($p < 0.001$) (positive predictive value = 0.71, negative predictive value = 0.62). A chi-square test excluding the severe OSA group showed that mild and moderate OSA groups did not show significance with respect to frequency of nocturnal voids. Kaynak H et al. Does frequency of nocturnal urination reflect the severity of sleep-disordered breathing? J Sleep Res 2004;13:173–176. Reprinted with permission from John Wiley & Sons, Inc

The clinical syndrome of OSA is defined as the combination of ≥5 apnea–hypopnea index (AHI) events/hour and significant self-reported sleepiness (the AHI is the sum of apneas and hypopneas during sleep divided by the sleep time in hours). The OSA syndrome is reported to affect around 2% of women and 4% of men [67]. Sleep apnea, as well as other common factors such as impaired arginine vasopressin secretion or reduced bladder capacity, can cause nocturnal polyuria, and in turn, nocturia, but nocturia is found at elevated levels only in those with severe OSA (>30 events/h; Fig. 3.8), and not in those with mild or moderate OSA [68].

Nocturnal polyuria in sleep apnea is evoked by negative intrathoracic pressure due to inspiratory effort against a closed or partially closed upper airway. Atrial natriuretic peptide (ANP) is released due to airway obstruction-related hypoxemia, which in turn causes pulmonary arterial constriction and an associated

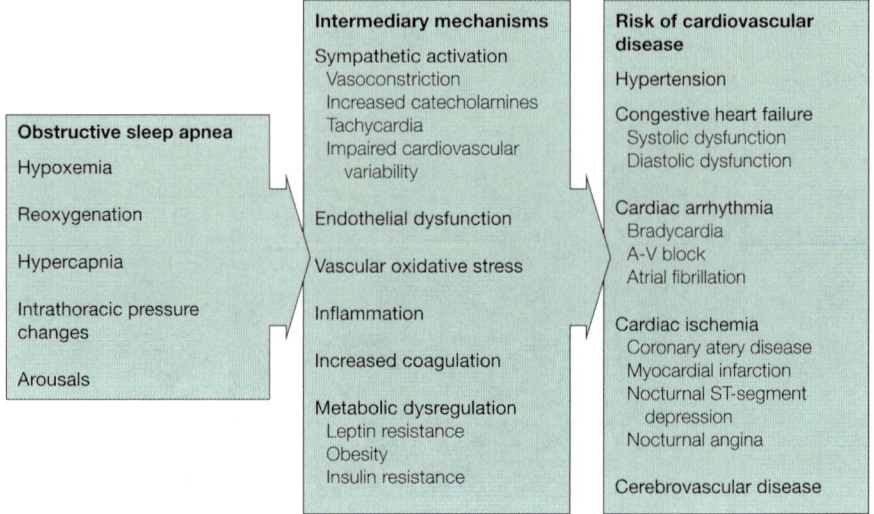

Fig. 3.9 Acute and intermediary mechanisms of OSA that contribute to risk of cardiovascular disease [71]. Abnormalities associated with obstructive sleep apnea (OSA) may be intermediary mechanisms that contribute to the initiation and progression of cardiac and vascular pathology. These mechanisms may interact with each other, thus potentiating their pathophysiological implications. Shamsuzzaman ASM et al. Obstructive sleep apnea: implications for cardiac and vascular disease. JAMA 290:1906–1914. Copyright © 2003 American Medical Association. All rights reserved

increase in right atrial pressure; the latter then secretes ANP in response [69]. This cardiac hormone increases sodium and water excretion, and also inhibits other hormone systems that regulate fluid volume, vasopressin, and the renin–angiotensin–aldosterone complex [70]. There are various possible sequelae of OSA, meaning that, like poor sleep itself, it can have serious consequences for health (Fig. 3.9) [71].

Diagnosis and Treatment of OSA

Many of the symptoms of sleep apnea, such as snoring and fatigue, are nonspecific. The American Academy of Sleep Medicine (AASM) guidelines advise "diagnostic criteria for OSA are based on clinical signs and symptoms determined during a comprehensive sleep evaluation, which includes a sleep-oriented history and physical examination, and findings identified by sleep testing" [72]. The two accepted methods of objective testing are in-laboratory polysomnography (PSG) and home testing with portable monitors (PM). A flowchart summarizing the recommended approach to OSA diagnosis and treatment is shown in Fig. 3.10.

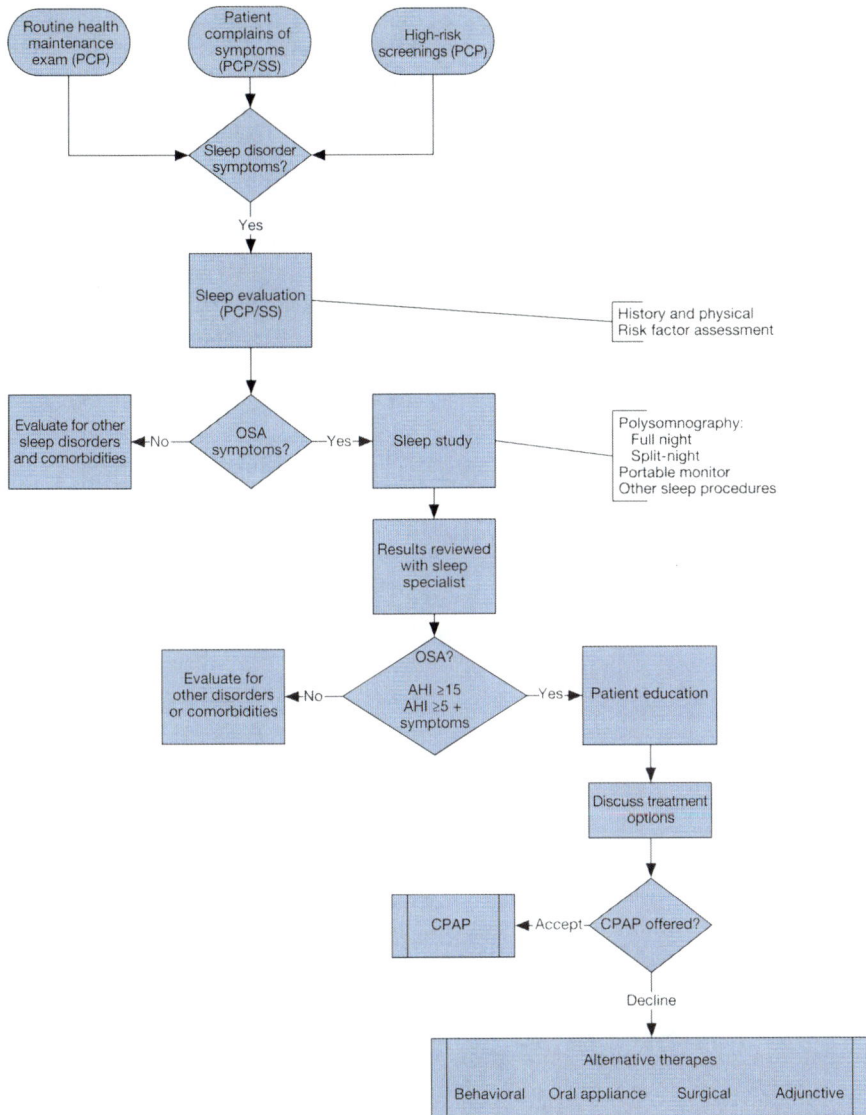

Fig. 3.10 Flowchart showing evaluation and treatment options for patients with suspected OSA [72]. *CPAP* continuous positive airway pressure, *OSA* obstructive sleep apnea, *PCP* primary care physician, *SS* sleep specialist. Epstein LJ et al. Clinical guideline for the evaluation, management and long-term care of obstructive sleep apnea in adults. J Clin Sleep Med 5(3):263–276. Copyright 2009 Reproduced with permission of American Academy of Sleep Medicine via Copyright Clearance Center

There are medical, behavioral, and surgical options for the treatment of OSA; positive airway pressure (PAP) is the recommended first-line treatment for mild, moderate and severe OSA, has been shown to reduce frequency of nocturnal voiding [73], and should be offered to all patients [72]. Alternative therapies may be offered depending on the severity of the OSA and the patient's anatomy, risk factors, and preferences. For a detailed description of OSA evaluation and treatment, see the AASM guidelines [72].

In a home sleep study, the prevalence of OSA was double among urogynecology patients with nocturia compared with those without [74]. However, in a population-based study by Tikkinen et al. [75], reported OSA was not associated with nocturia after adjustment, which may be due to the correlation with snoring, which represents partial negative pressure breathing (three-quarters of subjects with OSA reported snoring, and snoring was ten times more prevalent than OSA). Nonetheless, nocturia may be a result of OSA or other primary sleep disorders, such as insomnia or restless leg syndrome [76], and as such clinicians should thoroughly evaluate whether nocturia may be secondary to such conditions.

Nocturia-Related Sleep Deprivation: Costs to Society

Sleep disturbance – whether it be due to nocturia as a primary cause, to a primary sleep disorder or some other cause – is necessarily linked with a level of burden not only for the individual (QoL, health), but also to the family/caregiver (disruption to sleep), and to society (cost of reduced productivity, treatment of associated morbidity and injury).

Poor sleep imposes a significant socioeconomic burden as a consequence of the adverse effects of sleep disturbance on individual sufferers. The direct cost of insomnia (cost of medical care or self-treatment incurred by patients, healthcare providers or the government) was estimated to be $13.6 billion in the United States in 1995 [77]. Indirect costs are also a major contributor to the economic burden of poor sleep. A recent economic analysis concluded that indirect costs attributed to absenteeism and reduced work productivity accounted for 76% of the total cost of insomnia [78]. A retrospective claims-based study that examined the costs of untreated insomnia showed that both younger and older patients with insomnia incurred greater indirect and direct costs than those without insomnia [79].

There is limited published information available on the economic consequences of nocturia. A prospective Swedish study reported that overall work impairment (as assessed by the Work Productivity and Activity Impairment questionnaire) significantly increased as nocturia became more severe, and that those with nocturia had 9.2% greater overall work-impairment than controls [80]. This was estimated to represent an indirect cost of 9.2% of each affected individual's annual income. A recent analysis of the cost of nocturia (≥ 2 voids/night) in the United

States conservatively estimates the economic value of the productivity lost to be more than 60 billion USD annually and the medical cost of nocturia-associated falls in the elderly to be 1.5 billion USD [81]. A European analysis (≥3 voids/night) also highlights the significant economic burden of nocturia [82]. More studies in this area, to assess the economic burden represented by nocturia and by sleep disruption in nocturia, are needed.

Conclusions

Understanding the relationship between sleep and nocturia is important if therapies are to be developed to successfully treat these conditions. Although nocturia is consistently found to be the leading cause of sleep disturbance, it is important to recognize that there are no validated instruments that can reliably distinguish being awakened by the need to void as opposed to voiding out of convenience after one is awakened by something else. This distinction is critical to the understanding of the relationship between nocturia and sleep. As such, no study of sleep problems is complete without taking this common condition into consideration. Nocturia is associated with a wide range of negative outcomes, from poor functioning and QoL, to fractures, metabolic and endocrine disorders, and mortality. Our understanding of the mechanisms behind these relationships can be informed by the increasing body of sleep research demonstrating the critical role of sleep for our health and well-being (see Fig. 3.11), as well as recent studies aiming to dissect and delineate the impact of nocturia on specific sleep parameters. The importance of primary sleep disorders should also not be overlooked when diagnosing patients with nocturia, and nocturnal voiding should be managed according to its etiology. Evidence shows that nocturia is not a condition that can be ignored or considered merely "bothersome" or an inconvenience. Patients deserve thorough and strategic evaluation to ensure the best possible prognosis.

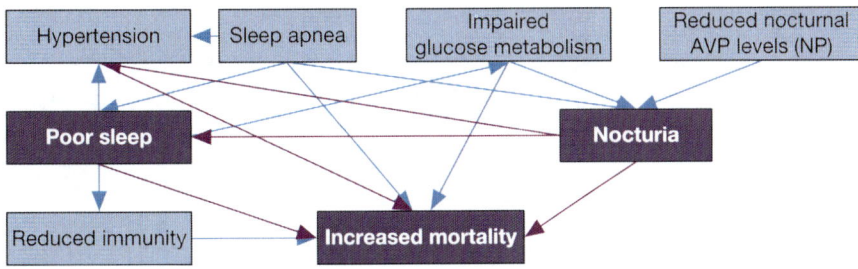

Fig. 3.11 Several possible factors in the complex relationship between nocturia, sleep, and health. *AVP* arginine vasopressin, *NP* nocturnal polyuria

Summary Points

- Mounting evidence demonstrates that nocturia is a predictor of mortality, independent of many comorbidities, in younger as well as older adults.
- Disruption to sleep which is caused by nocturia on a repeated basis may be an important mediator of the relationship between nocturia and poor health/mortality.
- The specific parameters of sleep, which are most significant for health are not yet known; however, adequate quantity and quality of sleep have both been shown to be critical for normal metabolic and endocrine functioning.
- Patients with nocturia may have reduced sleep quality (e.g., reduced sleep continuity, reduced SWS, reduced sleep efficiency), and possibly duration, which may contribute to poor QoL, increased falls, and reduced health and survival outcomes.
- Nocturia is not a benign condition – not only because of its effects on daytime functioning but also because it is a possible marker for increased morbidity and mortality.
- Nocturia is worthy of thorough medical evaluation in order to identify the cause in each affected individual (e.g., obstructive sleep apnea, nocturnal polyuria), and to proactively manage the condition.
- Further data are needed to investigate the impact of effective management of nocturia on long-term health outcomes.

References

1. Kupelian V, Rosen RC, Link CL, et al. Association of urological symptoms and chronic illness in men and women: contributions of symptom severity and duration–results from the BACH Survey. J Urol. 2009;181:694–700.
2. Asplund R. Mortality in the elderly in relation to nocturnal micturition. BJU Int. 1999;84: 297–301.
3. Nakagawa H, Niu K, Hozawa A, et al. Impact of nocturia on bone fracture and mortality in older individuals: a Japanese longitudinal cohort study. J Urol. 2010;184:1413–8.
4. Bursztyn M, Jacob J, Stessman J. Usefulness of nocturia as a mortality risk factor for coronary heart disease among persons born in 1920 or 1921. Am J Cardiol. 2006;98:1311–5.
5. Kupelian V, FitzGerald MP, Kaplan SA, Norgaard JP, Chiu GR, Rosen RC. Association of nocturia and mortality: results from the Third National Health and Nutrition Examination Survey. J Urol. 2011;185:571–7.
6. Ancoli-Israel S, Bliwise DL, Nørgaard JP. The effect of nocturia on sleep. Sleep Med Rev. 2011;15:91–7.
7. Yu HJ, Chen FY, Huang PC, Chen TH, Chie WC, Liu CY. Impact of nocturia on symptom-specific quality of life among community-dwelling adults aged 40 years and older. Urology. 2006;67:713–8.
8. Fiske J, Scarpero HM, Xue X, Nitti VW. Degree of bother caused by nocturia in women. Neurourol Urodyn. 2004;23:130–3.
9. Tikkinen KA, Johnson TM, Tammela TL, et al. Nocturia frequency, bother, and quality of life: how often is too often? A population-based study in Finland. Eur Urol. 2010;57:488–96.

10. Bliwise DL, Foley DJ, Vitiello MV, Ansari FP, Ancoli-Israel S, Walsh JK. Nocturia and disturbed sleep in the elderly. Sleep Med. 2009;10:540–8.
11. Spiegel K, Leproult R, Van CE. Impact of sleep debt on metabolic and endocrine function. Lancet. 1999;354:1435–9.
12. Gottlieb DJ, Punjabi NM, Newman AB, et al. Association of sleep time with diabetes mellitus and impaired glucose tolerance. Arch Intern Med. 2005;165:863–7.
13. Chao CY, Wu JS, Yang YC, et al. Sleep duration is a potential risk factor for newly diagnosed type 2 diabetes mellitus. Metabolism. 2011;60(6):799–804.
14. Spiegel K, Knutson K, Leproult R, Tasali E, Van Cauter E. Sleep loss: a novel risk factor for insulin resistance and Type 2 diabetes. J Appl Physiol. 2005;99:2008–19.
15. Gangwisch JE, Heymsfield SB, Boden-Albala B, et al. Sleep duration as a risk factor for diabetes incidence in a large U.S. sample. Sleep. 2007;30:1667–73.
16. Chaput JP, Després JP, Bouchard C, Astrup A, Tremblay A. Sleep duration as a risk factor for the development of type 2 diabetes or impaired glucose tolerance: analyses of the Quebec Family Study. Sleep Med. 2009;10:919–24.
17. Vgontzas AN, Liao D, Pejovic S, Calhoun S, Karataraki M, Bixler EO. Insomnia with objective short sleep duration is associated with type 2 diabetes: a population-based study. Diabetes Care. 2009;32:1980–5.
18. Cappuccio FP, D'Elia L, Strazzullo P, Miller MA. Quantity and quality of sleep and incidence of type 2 diabetes: a systematic review and meta-analysis. Diabetes Care. 2010;33:414–20.
19. Van CE, Knutson KL. Sleep and the epidemic of obesity in children and adults. Eur J Endocrinol. 2008;159 suppl 1:S59–66.
20. Gottlieb DJ, Redline S, Nieto FJ, et al. Association of usual sleep duration with hypertension: the Sleep Heart Health Study. Sleep. 2006;29:1009–14.
21. Vgontzas AN, Liao D, Bixler EO, Chrousos GP, Vela-Bueno A. Insomnia with objective short sleep duration is associated with a high risk for hypertension. Sleep. 2009;32:491–7.
22. Gangwisch JE. Epidemiological evidence for the links between sleep, circadian rhythms and metabolism. Obes Rev. 2009;10 suppl 2:37–45.
23. Staessen J, Bulpitt CJ, O'Brien E, et al. The diurnal blood pressure profile. A population study. Am J Hypertens. 1992;5:386–92.
24. Miller MA, Kandala NB, Kivimaki M, et al. Gender differences in the cross-sectional relationships between sleep duration and markers of inflammation: Whitehall II study. Sleep. 2009;32:857–64.
25. Meier-Ewert HK, Ridker PM, Rifai N, et al. Effect of sleep loss on C-reactive protein, an inflammatory marker of cardiovascular risk. J Am Coll Cardiol. 2004;43:678–83.
26. Preston BT, Capellini I, McNamara P, Barton RA, Nunn CL. Parasite resistance and the adaptive significance of sleep. BMC Evol Biol. 2009;9:7.
27. Kripke DF, Langer RD, Elliott JA, Klauber MR, Rex KM. Mortality related to actigraphic long and short sleep. Sleep Med. 2011;12:28–33.
28. Cappuccio FP, D'Elia L, Strazzullo P, Miller MA. Sleep duration and all-cause mortality: a systematic review and meta-analysis of prospective studies. Sleep. 2010;33:585–92.
29. Ancoli-Israel S, Klein B, Holm-Larsen T. Does the use of sleep questionnaires add to our knowledge about the impact of nocturia. Neurourol Urodyn. 2009;28:635–6.
30. Cai T, Gardener N, Abraham L, Boddi V, Abrams P, Bartoletti R. Impact of surgical treatment on nocturia in men with benign prostatic obstruction. BJU Int. 2006;98:799–805.
31. Aserinsky E, Kleitman N. Regularly occurring periods of eye motility, and concomitant phenomena, during sleep. Science. 1953;118:273–4.
32. Keenan SA. Normal human sleep. Respir Care Clin N Am. 1999;5:319–31.
33. Roehrs T. Sleep physiology and pathophysiology. Clin Cornerstone. 2000;2:1–15.
34. Stanley N. The underestimated impact of nocturia on quality of life. Eur Urol Suppl. 2005;4:17–9.
35. Ferrara M, De Gennaro L, Bertini M. Selective slow-wave sleep (SWS) deprivation and SWS rebound: do we need a fixed SWS amount per night? Sleep Res Online. 1999;2:15–9.

36. Diekelmann S, Born J. The memory function of sleep. Nat Rev Neurosci. 2010;11:114–26.
37. Ferrara M, De GL, Bertini M. The effects of slow-wave sleep (SWS) deprivation and time of night on behavioral performance upon awakening. Physiol Behav. 1999;68:55–61.
38. Plihal W, Born J. Effects of early and late nocturnal sleep on priming and spatial memory. Psychophysiology. 1999;36:571–82.
39. Landsness EC, Crupi D, Hulse BK, et al. Sleep-dependent improvement in visuomotor learning: a causal role for slow waves. Sleep. 2009;32:1273–84.
40. Dijk DJ. Regulation and functional correlates of slow wave sleep. J Clin Sleep Med. 2009;5(2 suppl):S6–15.
41. Lentz MJ, Landis CA, Rothermel J, Shaver JL. Effects of selective slow wave sleep disruption on musculoskeletal pain and fatigue in middle aged women. J Rheumatol. 1999;26:1586–92.
42. Toth LA. Sleep, sleep deprivation and infectious disease: studies in animals. Adv Neuroimmunol. 1995;5:79–92.
43. Toth LA, Tolley EA, Krueger JM. Sleep as a prognostic indicator during infectious disease in rabbits. Proc Soc Exp Biol Med. 1993;203:179–92.
44. Mullington J, Korth C, Hermann DM, et al. Dose-dependent effects of endotoxin on human sleep. Am J Physiol Regul Integr Comp Physiol. 2000;278:R947–55.
45. Haack M, Schuld A, Kraus T, Pollmacher T. Effects of sleep on endotoxin-induced host responses in healthy men. Psychosom Med. 2001;63:568–78.
46. Imeri L, Opp MR. How (and why) the immune system makes us sleep. Nat Rev Neurosci. 2009;10:199–210.
47. Tasali E, Leproult R, Ehrmann DA, Van CE. Slow-wave sleep and the risk of type 2 diabetes in humans. Proc Natl Acad Sci USA. 2008;105:1044–9.
48. Spiegel K, Tasali E, Leproult R, Van Cauter E. Effects of poor and short sleep on glucose metabolism and obesity risk. Nat Rev Endocrinol. 2009;5:253–61.
49. Sayk F, Teckentrup C, Becker C, et al. Effects of selective slow-wave sleep deprivation on nocturnal blood pressure dipping and daytime blood pressure regulation. Am J Physiol Regul Integr Comp Physiol. 2010;298:R191–7.
50. Blackwell T, Yaffe K, Ancoli-Israel S, et al. Poor sleep is associated with impaired cognitive function in older women: the study of osteoporotic fractures. J Gerontol A Biol Sci Med Sci. 2006;61:405–10.
51. Dam TT, Ewing S, Ancoli-Israel S, Ensrud K, Redline S, Stone K. Association between sleep and physical function in older men: the osteoporotic fractures in men sleep study. J Am Geriatr Soc. 2008;56:1665–73.
52. Cohen S, Doyle WJ, Alper CM, Janicki-Deverts D, Turner RB. Sleep habits and susceptibility to the common cold. Arch Intern Med. 2009;169:62–7.
53. Ohayon MM. Nocturnal awakenings and comorbid disorders in the American general population. J Psychiatr Res. 2008;43:48–54.
54. Asplund R, Aberg H. Nocturnal micturition, sleep and well-being in women of ages 40–64 years. Maturitas. 1996;24:73–81.
55. Dew MA, Hoch CC, Buysse DJ, et al. Healthy older adults' sleep predicts all-cause mortality at 4 to 19 years of follow-up. Psychosom Med. 2003;65:63–73.
56. Middelkoop HA, Smilde-van den Doel DA, Neven AK, Kamphuisen HA, Springer CP. Subjective sleep characteristics of 1,485 males and females aged 50–93: effects of sex and age, and factors related to self-evaluated quality of sleep. J Gerontol A Biol Sci Med Sci. 1996;51:M108–15.
57. Van Kerrebroeck P, Rezapour M, Cortesse A, Thuroff J, Riis A, Norgaard JP. Desmopressin in the treatment of nocturia: a double-blind, placebo-controlled study. Eur Urol. 2007;52:221–9.
58. Chartier-Kastler E, Leger D, Montauban V, Comet D, Haab F. Impact of nocturia on sleep efficiency in patients with benign prostatic hypertrophy. Prog Urol. 2009;19:333–40.
59. Stone KL, Ancoli-Israel S, Blackwell T, et al. Actigraphy-measured sleep characteristics and risk of falls in older women. Arch Intern Med. 2008;168:1768–75.
60. Stewart RB, Moore MT, May FE, Marks RG, Hale WE. Nocturia: a risk factor for falls in the elderly. J Am Geriatr Soc. 1992;40:1217–20.

61. Asplund R. Hip fractures, nocturia, and nocturnal polyuria in the elderly. Arch Gerontol Geriatr. 2006;43:319–26.
62. Parsons JK, Mougey J, Lambert L, et al. Lower urinary tract symptoms increase the risk of falls in older men. BJU Int. 2009;104:63–8.
63. Temml C, Ponholzer A, Gutjahr G, Berger I, Marszalek M, Madersbacher S. Nocturia is an age-independent risk factor for hip-fractures in men. Neurourol Urodyn. 2009;28:949–52.
64. Alvarez-Nebreda ML, Jimenez AB, Rodriguez P, Serra JA. Epidemiology of hip fracture in the elderly in Spain. Bone. 2008;42:278–85.
65. Carskadon MA. Sleep deprivation: health consequences and societal impact. Med Clin North Am. 2004;88:767–76.
66. Williamson AM, Feyer AM. Moderate sleep deprivation produces impairments in cognitive and motor performance equivalent to legally prescribed levels of alcohol intoxication. Occup Environ Med. 2000;57:649–55.
67. Kapur VK. Obstructive sleep apnea: diagnosis, epidemiology, and economics. Respir Care. 2010;55:1155–67.
68. Kaynak H, Kaynak D, Oztura I. Does frequency of nocturnal urination reflect the severity of sleep-disordered breathing? J Sleep Res. 2004;13:173–6.
69. Yalkut D, Lee LY, Grider J, Jorgensen M, Jackson B, Ott C. Mechanism of atrial natriuretic peptide release with increased inspiratory resistance. J Lab Clin Med. 1996;128:322–8.
70. Umlauf MG, Chasens ER. Sleep disordered breathing and nocturnal polyuria: nocturia and enuresis. Sleep Med Rev. 2003;7:403–11.
71. Shamsuzzaman AS, Gersh BJ, Somers VK. Obstructive sleep apnea: implications for cardiac and vascular disease. JAMA. 2003;290:1906–14.
72. Epstein LJ, Kristo D, Strollo Jr PJ, et al. Clinical guideline for the evaluation, management and long-term care of obstructive sleep apnea in adults. J Clin Sleep Med. 2009;5:263–76.
73. Margel D, Shochat T, Getzler O, Livne PM, Pillar G. Continuous positive airway pressure reduces nocturia in patients with obstructive sleep apnea. Urology. 2006;67:974–7.
74. Lowenstein L, Kenton K, Brubaker L, et al. The relationship between obstructive sleep apnea, nocturia, and daytime overactive bladder syndrome in women. Am J Obstet Gynecol. 2008;198:598–5.
75. Tikkinen KA, Auvinen A, Johnson TM, et al. A systematic evaluation of factors associated with nocturia–the population-based FINNO study. Am J Epidemiol. 2009;170:361–8.
76. Pressman MR, Figueroa WG, Kendrick-Mohamed J, Greenspon LW, Peterson DD. Nocturia. A rarely recognized symptom of sleep apnea and other occult sleep disorders. Arch Intern Med. 1996;156:545–50.
77. Culpepper L. Secondary insomnia in the primary care setting: review of diagnosis, treatment, and management. Curr Med Res Opin. 2006;22:1257–68.
78. Daley M, Morin CM, Leblanc M, Gregoire JP, Savard J. The economic burden of insomnia: direct and indirect costs for individuals with insomnia syndrome, insomnia symptoms, and good sleepers. Sleep. 2009;32:55–64.
79. Ozminkowski RJ, Wang S, Walsh JK. The direct and indirect costs of untreated insomnia in adults in the United States. Sleep. 2007;30:263–73.
80. Kobelt G, Borgstrom F, Mattiasson A. Productivity, vitality and utility in a group of healthy professionally active individuals with nocturia. BJU Int. 2003;91:190–5.
81. Holm-Larsen T, Weiss J, Langkilde K. Economic burden of nocturia in the US adult population. J Urol. 2010;183:e1.
82. van Kerrebroeck P, Holm-Larsen T. The cost of nocturia in Europe. Abstract 373 presented at ICS/IUGA 2010 (non-discussion poster).

Chapter 4
Diary-Based Population Analysis of Nocturia in Older Men: Findings of the Krimpen Study

Boris van Doorn and J.L.H. Ruud Bosch

Keywords Diary-based population analysis • Nocturia • Older men • Krimpen study • Frequency volume charts • Nocturnal polyuria • International Prostate Symptom Score (IPSS)

Introduction

Increased diurnal and nocturnal voiding frequency are common and bothersome symptoms in older men and interfere with daily activities, whereas nocturia may result in sleep disturbance, daytime fatigue, a lower level of general well-being, and is a risk factor for nightly falls [1]. In the FInnish National Nocturia and Overactive bladder (FINNO) study, health-related quality of life was not impaired when subjects voided once a night, but slightly or moderately impaired with two or three or more voids per night, respectively [2]. In addition to the association with urological conditions, such as prostate enlargement, diurnal and nocturnal urinary frequencies are reported as symptoms of various diseases [3]. Many physicians consider increased nocturnal voiding frequency a sign of increased nocturnal urine production, which may represent a pathologic condition reflective of congestive heart failure, venous stasis or hormonal changes with ageing. Besides the relation to nocturnal urine production, nocturnal voiding frequency has been described as a result of diuretic use and awakenings for other reasons such as sleep disorders or anxiety [3].

With growing attention to urologic problems and the increasing number of older men, it is expected that physicians will see more men with these problems.

According to the most recent ICS definition, *nocturia* is the number of voids recorded during a night's sleep: each void is preceded and followed by sleep [4].

B. van Doorn, MD (✉) • J.L.H.R. Bosch, MD, PhD
Department of Urology, University Medical Center Utrecht, Utrecht, The Netherlands
e-mail: b.vanDoorn@umcutrecht.nl

When evaluating these patients, physicians are hampered by a paucity of population-based data on normal voiding patterns and related factors. Mostly, normal voiding patterns have been determined with the use of questionnaires. Validated questionnaires are useful for recording symptoms, their frequency, severity and bother, as well as the impact of LUTS on QoL, but are generally influenced by recall bias [5]. Frequency–volume charts are not subject to this type of bias and, therefore, they are a more valid tool for measuring urinary frequency [6]. Reports on the agreement between chart data and questionnaires have been contradictory [7, 8].

According to the most recent ICS definition, *nocturnal polyuria* is present when an increased proportion of the 24-h output occurs at night [4]. Normally, the night is considered to be a period of about 8 h whilst the patient is in bed. A weakness of this definition is the fact that the time a person actually is in bed varies and depends on age. The ICS standardisation report on terminology further states that the *normal range of nocturnal urine production* differs with age and the normal range remains to be defined. Therefore, nocturnal polyuria is present when greater than 20% (young adults) to 33% (over 65 years) is produced at night. Hence, the precise definition is dependent on age [4]. Thus, normal values on nocturnal urine production and its relation to nocturnal frequency in older men were lacking before the analyses of the Krimpen study.

In general, previously suggested definitions of nocturnal polyuria, most of which refer to a day/night ratio in urine production, were not based on normal distributions and were not properly validated [9]. Also, the incidence of nocturia and nocturnal polyuria in the community needed to be studied.

Frequency Volume Charts

The ICS report on standardisation of terminology in lower urinary tract function defines a frequency volume chart as follows: a FVC records the volumes voided as well as the time of each micturition, day and night, for at least 24 h. This is usually commenced after the first void produced after rising in the morning and is completed by including the first void on rising the following morning [4]. We may add to this that for a proper analysis of nocturia and nocturnal polyuria, it is necessary that subjects record the time of going to bed and time of rising.

Why do FVCs give a better insight in the condition "nocturia" than studies based on questionnaire data? Clearly, FVCs [but not questionnaires] are excellent tools to evaluate nocturnal urine production in an epidemiological setting. Furthermore, the relationship between nocturia and [nocturnal] polyuria can only be explored using FVCs. As already stated, data derived from questionnaires like the International Prostate Symptom Score (IPSS) are prone to recall bias [5]. There are some differences between IPSS-based and FVC-based data that need further attention. The IPSS refers to a period of one month preceding the moment of completion of the questionnaire, whereas an FVC covers a period of at least 24 h but preferably 3 days. One might ask whether FVCs are therefore more prone to fluctuation than the

IPSS, when serially administered? Because of the burden of completing a FVC, the response rate may be lower. Inevitably, some subjects will complete the FVC incorrectly.

The following measurements can be abstracted from frequency volume charts:

1. Daytime voiding frequency: the number of voids recorded during waking hours; this includes the last void before sleep and the first void after waking and rising in the morning.
2. Nocturia: the number of voids recorded during a nights sleep: each void is preceded and followed by sleep.
3. 24-h voiding frequency is the total number of daytime voids and episodes of nocturia during a specified 24-h period.
4. 24-h urine production is measured by collecting all urine for 24 h.
5. The maximum voided volume (MVV) at daytime and at night (formerly often referred to as functional bladder capacity (FBC). The MVV is the largest volume of urine voided during a single micturition.

To our knowledge, the Krimpen study is the only community-based study that has used frequency–volume charts to determine normal voiding frequency values and voided volumes as well as their determinants in older community-dwelling men. The following have been studied and described:

The Krimpen Study Protocol

The Baseline Round

In the Krimpen study all 3,924 men aged 50–75 years residing in a Dutch municipality (Krimpen aan den IJssel) near Rotterdam were evaluated to gain information on the natural history of male lower urinary tract and genital tract dysfunction. Men without radical prostatectomy, prostate or bladder cancer, neurogenic bladder disease or negative advice from their general practitioner, who were able to complete questionnaires and attend the health centre, were invited for the study. The baseline round of the study consisted of phase 1, in which data of 1,688 responders (50% of all eligible men) were collected by way of self-administered 113-item questionnaires and during a visit to a primary care health centre and phase 2, in which 1,661 men (98.4% of the participants) visited a urology outpatient clinic.

The questionnaire included the International Prostate Symptom Score (IPSS) and questions on chronic disease history such as cardiovascular symptoms, hypertension and diabetes mellitus, smoking habits, alcohol consumption and current medication use.

Measurements at the health centre included: height, body weight, systolic and diastolic blood pressure, and urinalysis by a dipstick test. At the urology outpatient department, additional measurements were made: serum prostate specific antigen, digital rectal examination and transrectal prostatic ultrasound, uroflowmetry, and post-void residual urine volume. To exclude men with prostate carcinoma, biopsies were taken according to a PSA-driven protocol.

A 3-day frequency–volume chart was completed by 1,597 participants (95%), on which each micturition was recorded in one-hour time units. On day 3, each voided volume was recorded. The time of rising and bedtime were noted on the chart by the participants. Diurnal and nocturnal urinary frequencies were determined from the time of rising on the first day until time of rising on the third day. We estimated 24-h urinary frequency as the mean during three days, or two when one was missing. The number of voids during patient-reported waking and sleeping hours was estimated as the mean of two or the frequency of one day and night, respectively, when the other was missing. Voiding at the time of rising and just before bedtime was considered diurnal frequency. We defined nocturia as voiding for which sleep was interrupted and designated two or more, and three or more of such voids as, *nocturia* ≥ 2 and *nocturia* ≥ 3, respectively. Men with 1.5 and 2.5 voids in two nights on the frequency–volume chart were included in the *nocturia* ≥ 2 and *nocturia* ≥ 3 groups, respectively. The nocturnal urinary *volume* was determined from midnight until time of rising. The initial daytime voiding within one hour after rising was included into nocturnal urinary volume. Nocturnal polyuria was defined as nocturnal urinary volume greater than 35% of the 24-h total urine volume [9]. *Clinical BPH* was defined as having moderate to severe voiding symptoms (IPSS greater than 7 points) with prostate enlargement (volume greater than 30 cm^3) and a reduced urinary peak-flow rate (less than 15 ml per second) [10]. We compared the number of voids during patient-reported and arbitrarily defined sleeping hours: 11 p.m. to 7 a.m., 11 p.m. to 8 a.m., midnight to 7 a.m. or midnight to 8 a.m.

The ICS report on standardisation of terminology in lower urinary tract function defines *nocturnal urine volume* as the total volume of urine passed between the time the individual goes to bed with the intention of sleeping and the time of waking with the intention of rising [4]. Therefore, it excludes the last void before going to bed but includes the first void after rising in the morning. This consequently means that it includes urine that is produced between rising and the first void after rising and that it includes urine produced between the last void before going to bed and the time of going to bed. To correct for these errors, we computed urine production for each hour of the day according to the method described by Van Mastrigt and Eijskoot [11]: urine production was assumed to be constant between two voidings and hourly urine production was estimated as the volume of each micturition divided by the number of hours that passed since the previous micturition (Fig. 4.1). Nocturnal urine production was estimated as the mean hourly urine production (ml/h) from 1 a.m. to 6 a.m. This period was chosen because (approximately) 90% of the men were "asleep" in this period. Nocturnal voiding frequency was estimated using patient-reported sleeping times. A 24-h voided volume greater than 2,500 ml was arbitrarily defined as "24-h polyuria," although the ICS report on standardisation of terminology in lower urinary tract function defines *polyuria* as a measured production of more than 2.8 l of urine in 24 h in adults. The figure of 2.8 l is based on a 70 kg person voiding >40ml/kg.

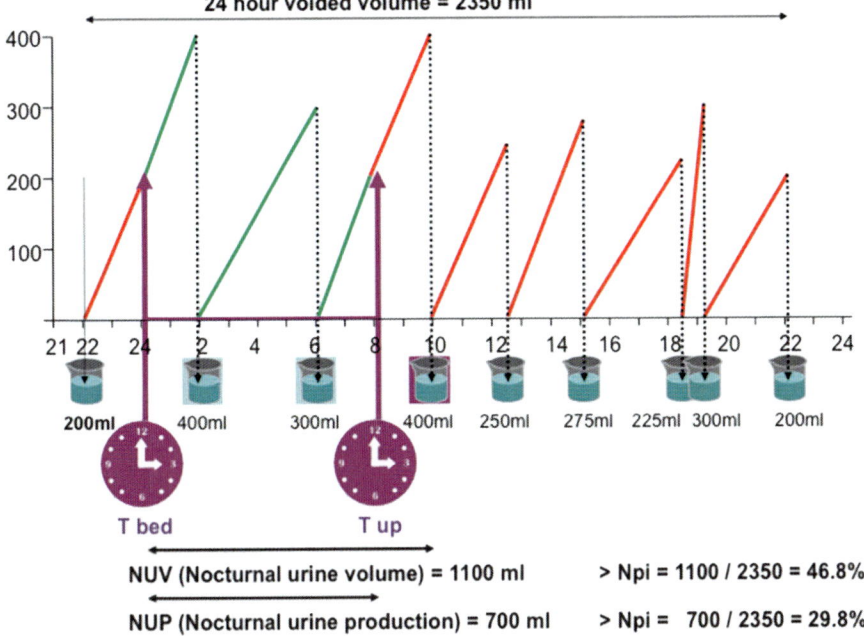

Fig. 4.1 Proper calculation of nocturnal urine production. Calculation according to the method of van Mastrigt and Eijskoot (see text) results in lower nocturnal polyuria index (Npi) than with the method suggested by ICS committee on standardisation of terminology (see text)

Participants were similar to those not responding for age, smoking and drinking habits and chronic diseases; participants more often had moderate to severe lower urinary tract symptoms [12].

Analysis of the Data

Men with newly diagnosed prostate cancer or previous operation for benign prostatic hyperplasia ($n = 106$) were excluded from the analyses because we primarily evaluated the natural history of lower urinary tract symptoms. Of the remaining men, 60 completed the frequency–volume chart inadequately and were therefore excluded; thus, 1,432 men constituted the basis for the cross-sectional baseline analysis. Certain determinants were entered into multivariate models individually, including age group, diabetes mellitus (yes or no), cardiovascular symptoms (yes or no), hypertension indicated by diastolic and systolic blood pressure greater than 94 and 159 mm Hg, respectively, or antihypertensive drug use, diuretic use (yes or no), alcohol consumption (no alcohol, 1–2 units per day or more than 2 units per day), smoking habits (yes or no), post void residual volume of >50 ml, nocturnal polyuria (yes or no), clinical BPH (yes or no), IPSS groups (no, mild, moderate or severe symptoms), prostate enlargement (yes or no) and reduced urinary peak flow rate (yes or no). To assess the possible effect of variables in the *nocturia* ≥ 2 and *nocturia*≥3 group, bivariate logistic regression for repeated measurements was done. In both the linear and logistic regression analyses, variables with a p-value <0.25 entered multivariate models with diurnal voiding frequency and nocturia as dependent variables. We tested two models: one with clinical BPH (model A) and one with IPSS, prostate enlargement and reduced urinary peak flow rate as separate parameters (model B). Final analyses were performed using variables with a p-value <0.05 in the multivariate models. Linear regression approach enabled us to estimate diurnal voiding frequency in men with a certain characteristic relative to those without this characteristic, while controlling for other factors. The logistic regression approach produced adjusted odds ratios (ORs), indicating the probability of nocturia in men with a certain characteristic in regard to a reference group, while controlling for other characteristics.

As a measure of agreement between responses to the IPSS question on nocturia and the frequency–volume chart data, we calculated the intra-class correlation. A correlation coefficient of 1 indicated perfect agreement; a correlation of zero indicates no agreement at all. A p-value of 0.05 was considered significant.

We also performed linear regression analyses on nocturnal urine production to explore possible determinants. In the analyses on the relation between urine production and voiding frequency, the latter is considered as the dependent variable, as changes in nocturnal urine production may lead to changes in nocturnal voiding frequency, rather than be a result of it. In these analyses, data of men that reported sleeping times ($n=1124$) are used. Nocturnal urine production did not differ between these men and those who did not report sleeping times (mean 60.2 and 61.4 ml/h, respectively).

We tested the value of nocturnal urine production in addition to the other previously described determinants of nocturnal voiding frequency. Different cut-off values of nocturnal urine production were added to the logistic regression models with these determinants. Moreover, we corrected for the number of sleeping hours reported by the individuals and tested the effect of bladder voiding efficiency on nocturnal voiding frequency. The model with the highest percentage of explained variance was determined as best model. For the cut-off value of nocturnal urine production in these best models, the test characteristics (true positive rate, TPR, and false positive rate, FPR) were derived from ROC curves.

The following measurements resulted from the cross-sectional analysis of the baseline data:

1. Age-group-specific normal values of diurnal and nocturnal voiding frequencies in older men.
2. The age-group-specific prevalence of nocturia.
3. Determinants of increased voiding frequency (such as urological parameters and general medical conditions).
4. The influence of the definition of sleeping hours on nocturnal frequency.
5. The level of agreement between frequency–volume chart and questionnaire data, regarding nocturia.
6. Normal values for nocturnal urine production in older men, based on recordings on frequency–volume charts.

7. The age-group-specific prevalence of nocturnal polyuria.
8. Determinants of nocturnal polyuria.
9. The association between nocturnal urine production and nocturnal voiding frequency.
10. A new definition of nocturnal polyuria was suggested.

The Follow-up Rounds

If no exclusion criteria were met, men were considered eligible for re-invitation for three subsequent follow-up rounds. These rounds were performed at 2.1, 4.2 and 6.5 years (mean), and included the questionnaire and the urology outpatient visit.

In each study round, the participants again completed a 3-day FV-chart. The percentage of men with a nocturnal voiding frequency of 2 or more (nocturia≥2) and 3 or more (nocturia≥3), respectively, was determined for 5-year age strata. Prevalence rates were estimated for each study round, separately. The possibility of normalising nocturnal frequency (i.e., having nocturia≥2 or nocturia≥3 in the first follow-up, but not in the second follow-up) is not ignored. The number of men available for analysis with adequate data in the final round was too small to perform adequate statistical analyses (mainly because time of rising and bedtime were missing). Therefore, for the *epidemiology of nocturia*, we present data from baseline and first (2.1 year) and second (4.2 year) follow-up round.

To study the *epidemiology of nocturnal polyuria*, urine production (UP) for each hour of the day was again determined as described above. Nocturnal UP (NUP) per hour was estimated as the mean between 1 am and 6 am, because 90% of the men were asleep in this period. This approach also solves the problem that a significant part of the participants did not accurately report the time of rising and bedtime. Three different definitions of nocturnal polyuria were used:

1. Nocturnal urine volume greater than 33% of 24-h total urine volume (abbreviated as "NUP33%/24h"; this is the most commonly used definition, in spite of theoretical and practical shortcomings).
2. NUP greater than 90 ml/h (abreviated as "NUP90"; previously suggested as a reasonable discriminator for nocturia (nocturia≥3) [13].

The percentage of men with nocturnal polyuria was determined for the different age strata using the three definitions. Prevalence rates of nocturnal polyuria (two definitions) were estimated for each study round.

The following measurements resulted from the longitudinal analysis of the follow-up rounds data:

1. The age-specific prevalence of nocturia in community-dwelling older men in the first (2.1 year) and second (4.2 year) follow-up round.
2. The age-specific prevalence of nocturnal polyuria in community-dwelling older men in the first (2.1 year) and second (4.2 year) follow-up round.

Findings of the Krimpen Study

Cross-Sectional Data [14]

A total of 1,597 men (95% of the responders) completed the 3-day frequency–volume chart. Two charts were excluded from analysis due to inadequate completion and 41 charts had missing values on one of the three days. Because of missing data on time of rising and bedtime, diurnal and nocturnal voiding was only estimated in 1,201 men (75% of the completed charts). The rate of missing values on time of rising and bedtime differed among age groups. It was highest and lowest in men aged 50–54 years and 70–78 years (43% and 18%, respectively). There were no differences in men with and without recorded waking and sleeping hours concerning 24-h voiding frequency and IPSS scores.

Figure 4.2 shows the circadian variation in urinary frequency during three days. Results in the three youngest and the two oldest age groups were similar. Therefore, the data were combined to age groups: 50–64 years and 65 years and older. Table 4.1 shows 24-h, diurnal and nocturnal voiding frequency in 5-year age groups. The mean duration of the sleeping time differed between the age groups. It was least and greatest in the 55–59- and 70–78-year-old groups (8.1 versus 8.6 h, analysis of variance test for trend, $p<0.001$). These differences were corrected as the number of voids per patient-reported sleeping hour.

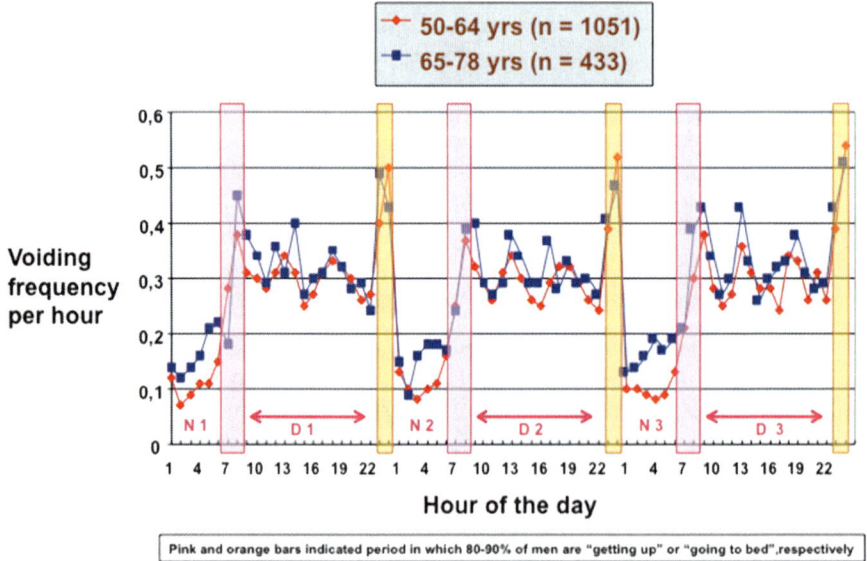

Fig. 4.2 Circadian variation in voiding frequency per hour of the day. Circadian variation is less clear in men over 65 years (*blue line*)

Table 4.1 Voiding frequency in population sample of men aged 50–78 years

Age group (years)	Voiding frequency			Number of voids per reported sleeping hour
	24-h frequency	Diurnal frequency	Nocturnal frequency	
50–54	5.7 (5.0–7.0)	5.0 (4.0–6.0)	1.0 (0.3–1.5)	0.11 (0–0.17)
55–59	6.0 (4.7–7.0)	5.0 (4.0–6.0)	1.0 (0–1.5)	0.13 (0–0.18)
60–64	6.3 (5.3–7.7)	5.0 (4.0–6.5)	1.0 (0.5–2.0)	0.13 (0.06–0.22)
65–69	6.5 (5.7–8.0)	5.0 (4.0–6.0)	1.5 (1.0–2.0)	0.16 (0.10–0.22)
70–78	7.0 (5.7–8.3)	5.0 (4.0–6.5)	1.5 (1.0–2.0)	0.18 (0.11–0.25)
All	6.3 (5.0–7.5)	5.0 (4.0–6.0)	1.5 (1.0–2.0)	0.13 (0.06–0.21)

Values are medians (interquartile ranges)

Bivariate linear regression revealed that certain variables had a significant positive correlation with mean diurnal voiding frequency, including clinical BPH, cardiovascular symptoms, hypertension, post-void residual of greater than 50 ml, IPSS, prostate enlargement and decreased maximum urinary flow. However, in the two multivariate models including these parameters, only clinical BPH and IPSS independently influenced *diurnal* urinary frequency. Men with clinical BPH voided a mean of 1.2 times more than those without clinical BPH (6.2 versus 5.0). Men with mild, moderate and severe symptoms voided a mean of 0.7, 2.0 and 2.5 more times, respectively, than men without symptoms who voided 4.5 times.

Figure 4.3 shows the percent of nocturnal voids for the 5-year age groups, as estimated by frequency–volume charts and the IPSS nocturia question. Frequency–volume charts indicated a higher percent of *nocturia ≥2 and nocturia ≥3* than the IPSS question.

Results of the logistic regression analyses on *nocturia ≥2* and *nocturia ≥3* groups indicate that each condition depended on age and the presence of BPH. Moreover, nocturnal polyuria was independently associated with *nocturia ≥3*, whereas it had no significant relation with *nocturia ≥2*. The opposite was true for diuretics use. The effect of age is greater for *nocturia ≥3*. Only 4% and 22% of men were adequately categorised when the arbitrarily defined sleeping hours of midnight to 7 a.m. and 11 p.m. to 8 a.m., respectively, were used for estimating nocturia. These times would have resulted in substantially different data on nocturnal voiding frequency.

A non-response study showed that the participants were comparable to non-responders with respect to age, educational and marital status and for smoking and drinking habits [12]. The participants had higher IPSS-scores and a slightly lower level of general well-being than the non-responders. This result may have caused overestimation of the diurnal and nocturnal voiding frequency indicated by the frequency–volume chart since a higher IPSS-score corresponded with increased diurnal frequency and higher nocturia odds ratios. These considerations indicate that normal values in the general population may be slightly lower than those in our sample. In the current study, clinical BPH and IPSS-voiding symptoms were the only two factors with an influence on diurnal-voiding frequency. Participant age, cardiovascular symptoms, hypertension, mean post-void residual urine volume,

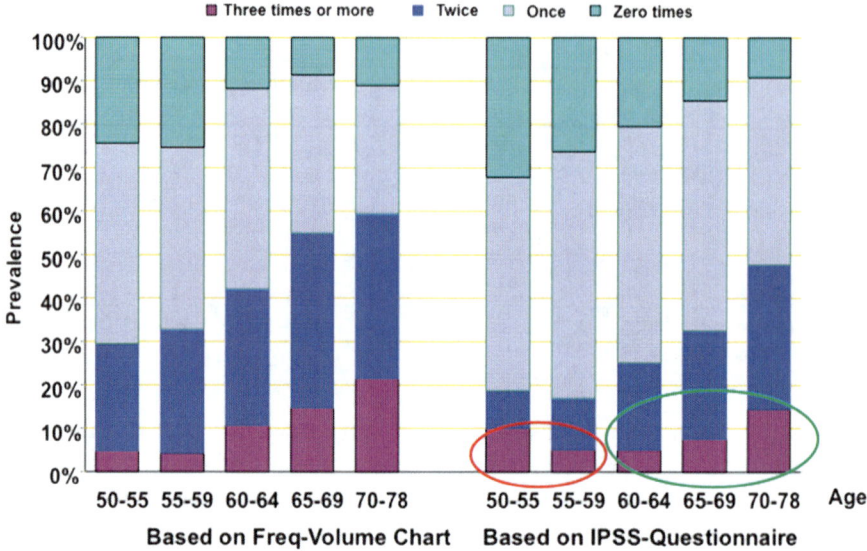

Fig. 4.3 Nocturnal voiding frequencies in community-dwelling men between 50 and 78 years, derived from frequency volume chart and questionnaire (IPSS nocturia question). In men below 60 years (*red oval*), the IPSS nocturia question overestimates the percentage with nocturia more than three times as compared to actual recordings on the frequency–volume chart. Men over 60 (*green oval*) underestimate their nighttime frequency when scoring the IPSS nocturia question

prostate enlargement and decreased maximum urinary flow did not influence diurnal frequency independent of these two factors. The present study shows that nocturia is common in older men, increasing strongly with increasing age (Fig. 4.3). The results of the Krimpen study also show a clear association of nocturia and clinical BPH, in community-dwelling older men.

Nocturnal polyuria is only associated with more severe nocturia, such as three voidings or more nightly. Diuretics use only has a role when there are two or more voids nightly. Although 28% of reports on "sleeping hours" were missing, we prefer the use of these patient-reported hours to the use of arbitrarily defined hours, because the latter method is highly inaccurate. Due to the lower number of missing reports on sleeping hours in elderly subjects, there was a relative over-representation of this group in the estimation of the nocturnal urinary frequency for the study population overall, which may have led to an overestimating of nocturia. We have no explanation for the significant difference in percentage of missing values on time of rising and bedtime between the young and old age group. We found a poor agreement of frequency–volume chart with questionnaire results.

The so-called "recognized determinants" of nocturia are based on *expert opinion* rather than scientific evidence: Ageing, BPH, depression, cardiovascular disease, life style factors, neurological disease (exclusion criterium for Krimpen study), nocturnal polyuria, bladder storage problems (e.g., overactive bladder), obesity, diabetes mellitus and sleep disorders.

In another large epidemiologic (questionnaire based) study, the FINNO study, the following determinants of nocturia were found in men: OAB, BPH and snoring, with less impact of obesity, antidepressant use, restless legs syndrome and prostate cancer [15]. In the Krimpen study, men with neurogenic bladder disease were not eligible and the 113-item questionnaire did not explore the presence of sleeping disorders, which clearly limits the possibility to study their role, although "snoring" is only a proxy of one type of sleeping disorder and cannot be reported by the subject himself who has to rely on the opinion of his partner. With these shortcomings in mind, we found that nocturia≥ 2 as well as nocturia≥ 3 groups depend on age and the presence of BPH. Moreover, nocturnal polyuria is independently associated with nocturia≥ 3, whereas it has no significant relation with nocturia-2. Diuretics use is only associated with nocturia≥ 2.

Mean nocturnal urine production was 60.6 ml/h (standard deviation 32.6) in men aged 50–78 years [13]. Univariate linear regression analyses yielded that alcohol consumption, body weight, post-void residual, number of sleeping hours, prostate enlargement and diabetes mellitus were non-significant ($p > 0.25$) determinants. In the multivariate analyses, the effect of hypertension, cardiac symptoms, reduced urinary flow rate and medication use was lost. The remaining significant determinants of increased nocturnal urine production (reference value: 53.4 ml/h for non-smoking men aged 50–54 years, without 24-h polyuria) based on multivariate analysis are: Age, smoking and 24-h polyuria.

Nocturnal urine production and nocturnal voiding frequency are clearly related, i.e., increased nocturnal voiding frequency is indicative of higher nocturnal urine production. This study indicates that nocturnal urine production is significantly higher in men with 24-h polyuria, which may result from habitually high fluid intake. Men who smoke have a slightly lower nocturnal urine production (−5.9 ml/h). Moreover, subclinical heart failure or venous stasis may be present more often in the older men (aged 65–78 years) than in the younger men (aged 50–64 years).

A cut-off value for increased nocturnal urine production was defined using logistic regression analysis. The best model was the one with the highest percentage of explained variance; and for the cut-off values of nocturnal urine production in these best models, the test characteristics (True positive rate [TPR] and false positive rate [FPR]) were derived from ROC curves. Using the cut-off value of 90 ml/h, 32% of the men with two or more voiding episodes would be classified correctly (true positive rate 0.32), whereas 6% of the men without two or more voiding episodes would be incorrectly classified (False positive rate 0.06). For three or more voiding episodes, the TPR and FPR are 0.46 and 0.12, respectively. Based on our analyses, we suggest that a nocturnal urine production exceeding 90 ml/h is abnormal. It should be stressed, however, that even this new definition predicts nocturnal voiding frequency only reasonably. Moreover, about one-third of the men with "increased" nocturnal urine production also have 24-h polyuria, most probably explaining the increased production.

In our opinion, future studies on medical treatment for "nocturnal polyuria" should first include patients with severe nocturia (e.g., nocturnal frequency of three times or more) and increased nocturnal urine production according to our new definition. In such studies, patients with 24-h polyuria, based on habitually excessive fluid intake, should be excluded. This suggestion is supported by a report of a phase III study on desmopressin in the treatment of nocturia in men [16]. In that study, it appeared that patients with nocturia who are treated for a polyuric factor respond better to treatment if nocturnal voiding frequency is three times or more.

Longitudinal Data

Nocturia Prevalence During Follow-up [17]

A total of 1,597 men (95% of responders) completed the 3-day FV-chart at baseline. Because of missing data on time of rising and bedtime, nocturnal voiding frequency could be estimated in 1,201 men (75% of the completed charts). The prevalence of men with nocturia≥2 and nocturia≥3 is presented in Table 4.2. The prevalence of nocturia≥2 and nocturia≥3 significantly increases over time for all age groups. The association with age was clear in all rounds, showing a higher prevalence of nocturia≥2 and nocturia≥3 with advancing age. There were 794 of 1,201 men without nocturia≥2 and 1,023 of 1,201 men without nocturia≥3 at baseline, respectively.

Nocturnal Polyuria Prevalence During Follow-up [18]

A total of 1,597 men (95% of responders) completed the 3-day FV-chart at baseline. Because of missing data, i.e., inadequately completed FV-charts, baseline nocturnal polyuria prevalence could be estimated in 1,532 men (96% of the completed charts). The prevalence of nocturnal polyuria for 5-year age strata, according to the two definitions, is shown in Table 4.3. For each definition, a clear relation with advancing age was shown. The lowest prevalence was shown for the definition NUP90, which was previously shown to be the best determinant of increased nocturnal voiding *frequency*. The longitudinal evolution of the prevalence rates in the subsequent study rounds only showed slight variations over time for all definitions. The largest increase over time (from 47.5% to 62.5%) was shown for NUP33%/24h in men from the baseline age stratum of 60–64 years.

At baseline, 454 of 1,532 men had no nocturnal polyuria according to the 33% definition (NUP33%/24h); 784 of 1,532 men had no NUP54; 1288 of 1,532 men had no NUP90.

The prevalence of nocturia [17] increases with age in a cross-sectional view at baseline; e.g., 2.8% of the men between 50–54 years, but 12.5% of the men between 65–69 years have Nocturia≥3. Furthermore, longitudinally, during the 4.2-year

Table 4.2 Prevalence of nocturia

Baseline age (years) strata	Baseline		2.1-year follow-up		4.2-year follow-up	
	Prevalence (n=1201)	(95% C.I.)	Prevalence (n=929)	(95% C.I.)	Prevalence (n=409)	(95% C.I.)
(a) Prevalence of nocturia two times or more						
50–54	20.1%	(14.7–25.5)	19.7%	(13.8–25.6)	41.5%	(29.2–53.8)
55–59	23.8%	(19.4–28.6)	29.2%	(23.4–35.1)	44.4%	(35.1–53.6)
60–64	34.1%	(28.7–39.6)	44.0%	(37.8–50.3)	61.3%	(52.1–70.5)
65–69	45.9%	(39.5–52.4)	45.5%	(38.1–52.9)	66.3%	(55.7–76.8)
70–78	54.9%	(46.9–62.9)	57.5%	(47.3–67.6)	65.8%	(50.0–81.6)
(b) Prevalence of nocturia three times or more						
50–54	2.8%	(0.6–5.0)	3.7%	(0.7–6.1)	7.7%	(1.0–14.4)
55–59	4.2%	(1.9–6.4)	5.1%	(2.3–7.9)	14.8%	(8.2–21.4)
60–64	7.9%	(4.8–11.1)	9.9%	(6.1–13.7)	17.1%	(10.0–24.2)
65–69	12.5%	(8.2–16.7)	18.5%	(12.8–24.3)	26.3%	(16.4–36.1)
70–78	17.0%	(11.0–23.0)	27.7%	(18.5–36.9)	28.9%	(13.8–44.1)

C.I. confidence interval

Table 4.3 Prevalence of nocturnal polyuria

Baseline age (years) strata	Baseline		2.1 year-follow-up		4.2-year follow-up		6.5-year follow-up	
	Prevalence ($n=1532$)	(95% C.I.)	Prevalence ($n=1080$)	(95% C.I.)	Prevalence ($n=803$)	(95% C.I.)	Prevalence ($n=739$)	(95% C.I.)
(a) Prevalence of nocturnal polyuria defined as NUP33%/24 h								
50–54	41.8%	(36.2–47.4)	44.3%	(37.4–51.2)	52.2%	(44.4–59.9)	51.4%	(44.0–58.9)
55–59	44.3%	(39.3–49.3)	44.2%	(38.4–50.1)	48.9%	(42.3–55.5)	48.8%	(42.1–55.6)
60–64	47.5%	(42.4–52.5)	48.8%	(42.9–54.6)	50.0%	(43.2–56.9)	62.5%	(55.4–69.6)
65–69	56.7%	(51.0–62.3)	54.2%	(47.3–61.0)	66.2%	(58.4–74.0)	65.3%	(56.7–73.9)
70–78	56.9%	(49.5–64.3)	66.4%	(57.5–75.2)	64.1%	(52.0–76.1)	59.1%	(44.0–74.2)
(b) Prevalence of nocturnal polyuria defined as NUP of >90 ml/h								
50–54	12.1%	(8.4–15.9)	14.3%	(9.4–19.1)	19.0%	(12.9–25.1)	19.0%	(13.1–24.9)
55–59	12.0%	(8.7–15.3)	11.6%	(7.8–15.3)	16.1%	(11.3–21.0)	17.2%	(12.1–22.3)
60–64	13.2%	(9.8–16.7)	20.1%	(15.3–24.8)	15.4%	(10.4–20.3)	25.7%	(19.3–32.1)
65–69	20.5%	(15.9–25.2)	19.7%	(14.2–25.2)	19.7%	(13.1–26.3)	20.8%	(13.5–28.2)
70–78	23.6%	(17.2–29.9)	23.0%	(15.1–30.9)	21.0%	(10.6–31.4)	25.6%	(12.0–39.2)

follow-up, the prevalence of nocturia per 5-year age stratum more than doubles for Nocturia≥3 [2.1–3.5 times] in men between 50 and 70 years at baseline. The prevalence of Nocturia≥2 increases less dramatically [1.4–2.0 times]. This increase is mainly due to increasing age of the baseline age strata (on average 4.2 years). Normalisation of nocturnal frequency can theoretically occur spontaneously, but also as a result of treatment (e.g., for cardiovascular disease or for LUTS). Subsequent analyses, linking this information with info from the charts/files of the general practitioners and pharmacy data, will resolve this problem.

The prevalence of NUP33%/24 h and NUP90 in community-dwelling men between 50 and 78 years clearly increases with age [18]. The prevalence rate of men with NUP33%/24 h is high (>40%) for all age strata; this indicates that this cut-off/definition can probably not be used as the only factor to determine whether a man needs treatment for this problem. The cross-sectional prevalence rate of NUP>90 ml/h increases from 12.1% between 50 and 54 to 23.6% between 70 and 78 years of age, also showing a clear age-related trend.

Analysis of the longitudinal data also shows that the prevalence per baseline age category increases somewhat. This is due to increasing age of the baseline age strata (on average 6.5 yrs). This means for example, that the prevalence of NUP33%/24h for the 50–54 year age stratum is 51.4% after 6.5 yrs of follow-up which is within the 95% CI of the baseline prevalence of the 60–64 year stratum (Table 4.3a). Normalisation of nocturnal polyuria can theoretically occur not only spontaneously but also as a result of some form of inter-current treatment (e.g., for cardiovascular disease or changes in drinking behaviour). Subsequent analysis linking this information with info from the charts of the general practitioners and pharmacy data will resolve this problem.

After adjustment for confounding variables, "lost to follow-up (LTFU)" in the first and second follow-up rounds was not related to LUTS severity, as measured by the IPSS. It is therefore unlikely that a selective LTFU, with a possible effect on prevalence rates, has occurred [19].

It is clear that nocturia is a multi-factorial condition with nocturnal polyuria as an important determinant; however, the age dependance of the functional bladder capacity (FBC) is another important factor that has to be taken into account. FBC is clearly related to LUTS in general. In Fig. 4.4, the relation between the presence of LUTS (IPSS>7) or the individual symptoms of the IPSS and the functional bladder capacity (FBC; defined as the largest single-voided volume recorded on the frequency–volume chart) is shown. Nocturia more than three times is more prevalent in men with lower FBC. However, average volumes per void as recorded on frequency–volume charts are significantly lower than FBC, indicating that men often void before FBC is reached and that sensory processing of the filling state is an additional factor determining the voided volumes.

The association among incident nocturnal polyuria and incident nocturia and the (evolving) functional bladder capacity is an interesting area for further study. Knowledge of the relative contributions of these elements will help to make better treatment choices for patients with bothersome nocturia and nocturnal polyuria. In some men, combination treatment might be appropriate for this condition.

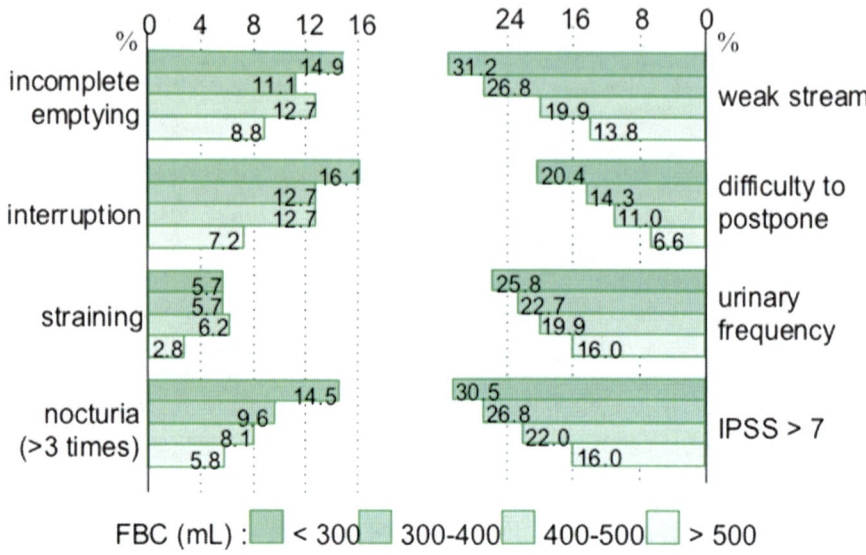

Fig. 4.4 Relation between the presence of LUTS (IPSS > 7) or the individual symptoms of the IPSS and the functional bladder capacity (FBC) defined as the largest single voided volume recorded on the frequency volume chart. Nocturia three times or more is more prevalent in men with lower FBC

Key Points

- In community-dwelling men aged 50–78 years, diurnal voiding frequency is higher in subjects with clinical BPH, whereas age has no influence.
- In community-dwelling men aged 50–78 years, nocturnal voiding frequency has a strong positive relation with age, clinical BPH, diuretics use and nocturnal polyuria, but does not seem to be associated with cardiovascular symptoms, diabetes mellitus or hypertension.
- Questionnaires underestimate the prevalence of nocturia, as compared to frequency–volume charts. In individual men, there is a lack of agreement between subjective (questionnaire and history taking) and objective prospectively collected (frequency–volume chart) data on nocturnal voiding frequency.
- The Krimpen study in community-dwelling men aged 50–78 years provides normal values and determinants for nocturnal urine production. Mean nocturnal urine production was 60.6 ml/h and increased considerably with advancing age and 24-h polyuria (smoking has a small additional effect).
- In community-dwelling men aged 50–78 years, the nocturnal voiding frequency is, on average, indicative of nocturnal urine production. However, nocturnal urine production is an only modest discriminator for increased nocturnal frequency.
- Based on analyses of frequency–volume charts in community-dwelling men aged 50–78 years, we suggest that a nocturnal urine production exceeding 90 ml/h is abnormal.

References

1. Asplund R, Aberg H. Health of the elderly with regard to sleep and nocturnal micturition. Scand J Prim Health Care. 1992;10:98–104.
2. Tikkinen KAO, Johnson II TM, Tammela TLJ, Sintonen H, Haukka J, Huhtala H, et al. Nocturia frequency, bother and quality of life: how often is too often? A population-based study in Finland. Eur Urol. 2010;57:488–98.
3. Barker JC, Mitteness LS. Nocturia in the elderly. Gerontologist. 1998;28:99–104.
4. Abrams P, Cardozo L, Fall M, Griffiths D, Rosier P, Ulmsten U, et al. The standardisation of terminology in lower urinary tract function; Report from the Standardisation Sub-committee of the International Continence Society. Neurourol Urodyn. 2002;21(2):167–78.
5. Coughlin SS. Recall bias in epidemiologic studies. J Am Epidemiol. 1990;43:87–91.
6. Abrams P, Klevmark B. Frequency volume charts: an indispensable part of lower urinary tract assessment. Scand J Ural Nephrol Suppl. 1996;179:47–53.
7. McCormack M, Infante-Rivard C, Schick E. Agreement between clinical methods of measurement of urinary frequency and functional bladder capacity. Br J Urol. 1992;69:17–21.
8. Donovan JL, Abrams P, Peters TJ, et al. The ICS – 'BPH' Study: the psychometric validity and reliability of the ICSmale questionnaire. Br J Urol. 1996;77:554–62.
9. Weiss JP, Blaivas JG. Nocturia. J Urol. 2000;163:5–12.
10. Bosch JL, Hop WC, Kirkels WJ, Schroder FH. Natural history of benign prostatic hyperplasia: appropriate case definition and estimation of its prevalence in the community. Urology. 1995;46:34–40.
11. van Mastrigt R, Eijskoot F. Analysis of voided urine volumes measured using a small electronic pocket balance. Scand J Urol Nephrol. 1996;30:257–63.
12. Blanker MH, Groeneveld FPMJ, Prins A, et al. Strong effects of definition and nonresponse bias on prevalence rates of clinical benign prostatic hyperplasia: the Krimpen study of male urogenital tract problems and general health status. BJU Int. 2000;85:665–71.
13. Blanker MH, Bernsen RMD, Bosch JLHR, Thomas S, Groeneveld FPMJ, Prins A, et al. Relation between nocturnal voiding frequency and nocturnal urine production in older men. Urology. 2002;60:612–6.
14. Blanker MH, Bohnen AM, Groeneveld FPMJ, Bernsen RMD, Prins A, Bosch JLHR. Normal voiding patterns and determinants of increased diurnal and nocturnal voiding frequency in elderly men. J Urol. 2000;164:1201–5.
15. Tikkininen KAO, Auvinen A, Johnson II TM, Weiss JP, Keränen T, Tiitinen A, et al. A systematic evaluation of factors associated with nocturia – the population based FINNO study. Am J Epidemiol. 2009;170:361–8.
16. Abrams P, Weiss J, Mattiasson A, et al. The efficacy and safety of oral desmopressin in the treatment of nocturia in men. Neurourol Urodyn. 2001;20:456–7.
17. van Doorn B, Blanker M, Bosch R. The incidence and prevalenceof nocturia (increased nocturnal voiding frequency): results from a community based study in older men. Neurourol Urodyn. 2009;28:928–30.
18. van Doorn B, Blanker M, Bosch R. The epidemiology of nocturnal polyuria (incidence and prevalence): a longitudinal community based study in men between 50 and 78 years of age. Neurourol Urodyn. 2009;28:765–6.
19. Blanker MH, Prins J, Bosch JLHR, Schouten BW, Bernsen RM, Groeneveld FP, et al. Loss to follow-up in a longitudinal study on urogenital tract symptoms in Dutch older men. Urol Int. 2005;75:30–7.

Chapter 5
Epidemiology of Nocturia: Evaluation of Prevalence, Incidence, Impact and Risk Factors

Kari A.O. Tikkinen, Theodore M. Johnson II, and Rufus Cartwright

Keywords Benign prostatic hyperplasia (BPH) • Lower urinary tract symptoms (LUTS) • Finnish National Nocturia and Overactive Bladder (FINNO) • Incidence of nocturia • Impact of nocturia • International Consultation on Incontinence Modular Questionnaire–Nocturia Quality of Life questionnaire • Reproductive factors in women

A Note on Definitions and Terminology

Until recently, nocturia has been a neglected topic in the medical literature [1], with early epidemiological research on urinary symptoms focussed either on lower urinary tract symptoms (LUTS) suggestive of benign prostatic hyperplasia (BPH) in men or on stress urinary incontinence in women. Within the last decade, nocturia has been recognised as a clinical entity in its own right [2, 3], leading to a resurgence of research interest (Fig. 5.1).

The definition of a symptom or condition is a critical factor in evaluating its epidemiology; nocturia is no exception to this rule [4]. Although our conception of

---

K.A.O. Tikkinen, MD, PhD (✉)
Department of Urology and Department of Clinical Epidemiology and Biostatistics,
Helsinki University Central Hospital, University of Helsinki, Helsinki, Finland

McMaster University, Hamilton, ON, Canada
e-mail: kari.tikkinen@fimnet.fi

T.M. Johnson II, MD, MPH
Emory University/Atlanta VA Medical Center,
Geriatric Medicine and Gerontology, Atlanta, GA, USA

R. Cartwright, MRCOG, MD(Res)
Queen Charlotte's and Chelsea Hospital, Institute of Reproductive
and Developmental Biology, Du Cane Road, London, UK

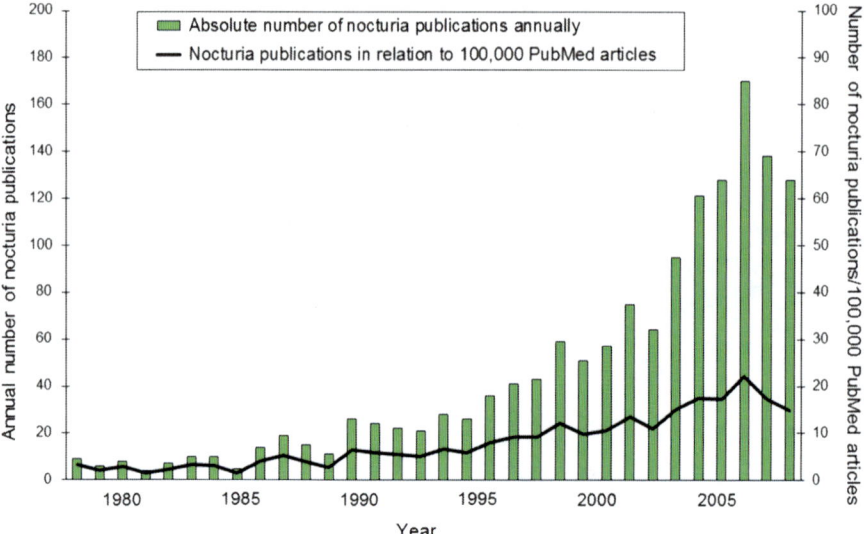

Fig. 5.1 Absolute and relative number of annual nocturia articles between 1978 and 2009. Separately for each time period (e.g., from Jan 1st, 1978 to Dec 31st, 1978), PubMed search was performed using word "nocturia" as search key. Number of annual publications was examined for the same time period. Updated from [11]

nocturia continues to evolve, working with standard definitions is vital to facilitate discussion and comparison between research studies. The International Continence Society classifies nocturia as one of the urinary storage symptoms and defines nocturia as "[t]he complaint that the individual has to wake at night one or more times to void…each void is preceded and followed by sleep" [3]. The updated International Urogynaecological Association/International Continence Society 2010 gender-specific standardisation report [5] modifies this definition to the "complaint of interruption of sleep one or more times because of the need to micturate," specifying also that "each void is preceded and followed by sleep." The National Institutes of Health (in the United States) Terminology Workshop for Researchers in Female Pelvic Floor Disorders provides a simpler definition [6] of "awakening from sleep to pass urine." The issue of having to go back to sleep afterwards would seem to be unnecessary. The intention of going back to sleep after voiding might be more clinically relevant. Perhaps the definition does not need to include this issue at all [7]. However, for practical purposes, it might be necessary to distinguish a nocturic void from the first void after rising. Overall, these idealised definitions are conceptually easy to use, but their ambiguity makes them difficult to apply in practice. They do not define nocturia by the severity or symptom bother and provide no information as to when nocturia becomes clinically meaningful and worthy of evaluation and treatment [8, 9]. A single nighttime void would meet criteria for nocturia by either definition, and yet there is a lack of evidence that it is a suitable criterion for clinical purposes.

Prevalence

Prevalence is a measure of the total number of cases of a condition in a population, whereas incidence is the rate of occurrence of new cases. Thus, prevalence indicates how widespread a condition is whereas incidence conveys information about the risk of the condition. As nocturia is a fluctuating symptom [10], not "irreversible" such as a cancer diagnosis, incidence figures can only be understood in context with information on remission. For many purposes, it is therefore unclear whether prevalence or incidence data are more relevant [11].

Reported estimates of the prevalence of nocturia have varied, largely due to differences in symptom assessment, study population, data collection and definitions used [4, 11]. Most earlier studies on nocturia prevalence were conducted among elderly men [12–17]. These studies found that nocturia increases with age and is a very common symptom in the elderly. Parallel results were also found in studies conducted among women [18–20].

There has been a paucity of studies assessing LUTS and/or nocturia in both sexes (with wide age range), especially using population-based samples. However, a number of comparative studies have confirmed the strong impact of ageing on prevalence of nocturia [8, 21–30].

In the population-based Finnish National Nocturia and Overactive Bladder (FINNO) Study of both sexes aged 18 to 79, approximately 40% of subjects reported voiding at least once per night after age standardisation (Fig. 5.2). With nocturia defined as at least two voids per night, approximately one out of eight men and women had nocturia [8]. Overall, nocturia was equally common among both sexes; however, in more detailed age-specific analyses, clear differences between the sexes emerged. Young women (18–29 years) reported over 10 times more nocturia than young men, whereas in older age groups men had more nocturia than women [8]. The rate of nocturia in men and women equalised only in the sixth to seventh decade of life. At the age of 50–59 years, approximately 11% of men and 15% of women voided at least twice per night. Among those aged 60–69, approximately 37% of men and 22% of women voided at least twice per night. At ages 70–79 years, approximately 44% of men and 34 % of women voided at least twice per night (Fig. 5.2) [11].

In the FINNO Study, the prevalence of nocturia (defined as at least one void/night) increased at a constant rate with age (Fig. 5.2). The mean increases in odds ratio (OR) were 7.3% (6.5–8.2%) per year for men and 3.5% (2.9–4.1%) per year for women. Thus, the increase in OR was over twice as high in men compared with women. The trend was also similar when nocturia was defined as at least two voids per night [8].

Many other recent studies have supported these findings of a higher prevalence of nocturia among young women than young men, and an equalisation of prevalence in middle age [27–32]. As the gender difference has been found across different continents (Europe, Asia, Australia and North America), it is probably not due to a specific country, lifestyle or culture (Fig. 5.3) [8, 11, 21, 27–31, 33]. The reasons for the excess of nocturia among young women remain unknown, but greater

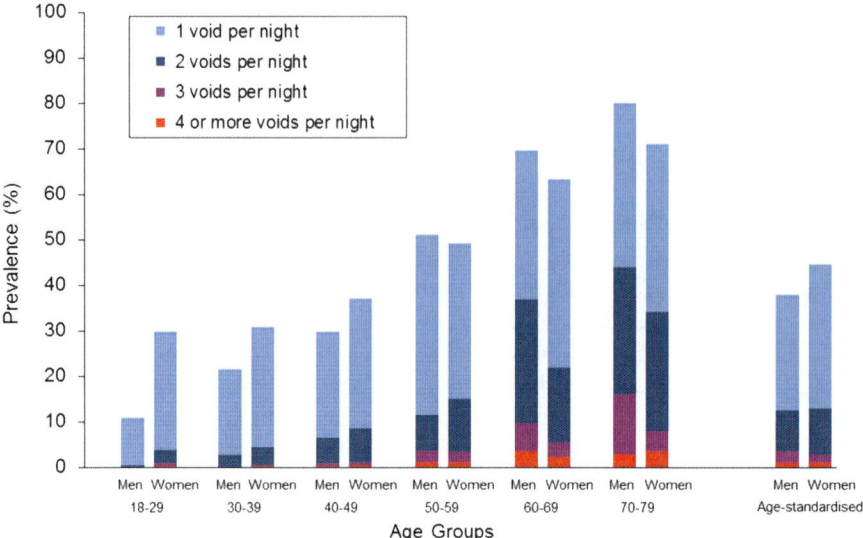

Fig. 5.2 Prevalence (%) of nocturia episodes by age group and gender in the FINNO Study, Finland, 2003–2004. Pregnant and puerperal women and those subjects reporting urinary tract infection were excluded. Age standardisation performed using the age structure of Finland (beginning of 2004). Modified from [11]

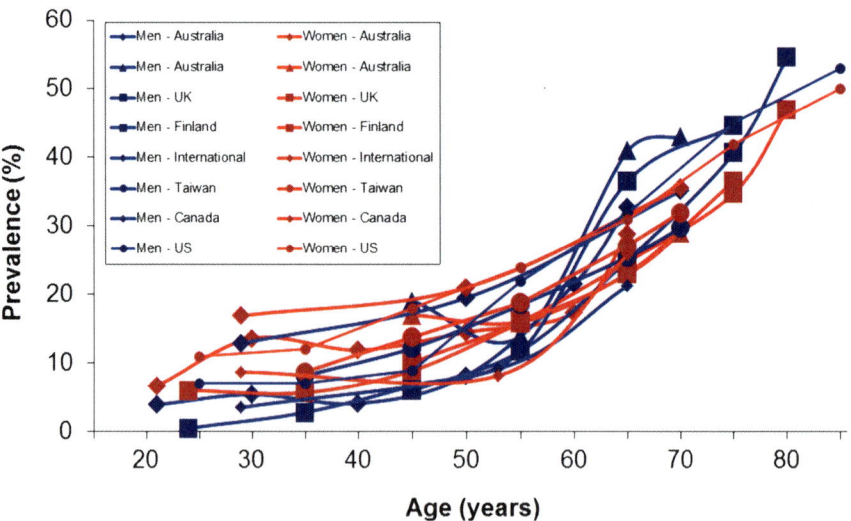

Fig. 5.3 Prevalence of at least two voids per night across age groups by sex in population-based studies conducted among both sexes with wide age range. Population-based studies (published in English before January 2011) with percentage data available conducted among both sexes with age range of at least 40 years were included [8, 11, 21, 27–31, 33]

fragmentation of sleep due to other causes and proneness to insomnia has been suggested [9]. At the other end of the age scale, the impact of prostate enlargement is likely to be the predominant factor in elderly men.

Questionnaire Versus Frequency–Volume Chart in Assessment of Nocturia Prevalence

Most earlier studies have used questionnaires for assessment of nocturia episodes. According to questionnaire studies, most elderly people void at least once per night [9]. In the Krimpen study [34], nocturia was assessed by frequency–volume charts (voiding diary). At least 1.5 voids per night (calculated based on information on two or three nights) was present in 30% of men aged 50–54 and in 60% of men aged 70–78 years, whereas at least 2.5 voids per night was present in 4% and 20%, respectively. These estimations are comparable to questionnaire studies (Figs. 5.2–5.3).

Whether frequency–volume charts or questionnaires provide more reliable information on population prevalence of nocturia, remain unknown. Undoubtedly, questionnaires are vulnerable to recall bias: questionnaires rely on the subject's memory. Subjects can forget an event entirely or forget the timing. Increasing concordance of questionnaire recall and voiding diaries has been found among those with few nocturia episodes (0, 1 or 2 voids/night) [35, 36]. Those are the critical episodes that determine the clinical impact of nocturia, which clearly enhances the usability of questionnaires. Theoretically, the use of voiding diaries should not only provide greater accuracy but also include information on nocturnal polyuria (i.e., overproduction of urine at night). However, in real-life (epidemiological) research, one should take into account that the use of frequency–volume charts compared to questionnaires has substantial methodological risks. There may be increased risk of selection bias (due to probable recruitment problems), with a lower response proportion and/or unrepresentative study population. In addition, the remarkable variation in nocturnal voiding [36] may not be captured by frequency–volume charts typically lasting only one to three nights. A questionnaire retrospectively assessing "the typical frequency" over a longer time period may be more representative. Finally, there is a possible impact of prospective evaluation itself on nocturnal voiding habits including a bladder-training effect [11, 37], and considerable sleep disruption associated with diary completion [38].

Incidence of Nocturia

While nocturia prevalence has been often well detailed [11], the literature on the incidence of nocturia remains relatively sparse in comparison. The reasons for this merit consideration.

Given how incidence studies must be performed, one realises immediately obvious concerns about how to meaningfully execute such a study. Accounting for the relative lack of data on nocturia incidence are several factors: the ready availability of cross-sectional data compared to longitudinal data [11]; the relative youth of recognition of and standardised definition for nocturia [3]; considerations about remission and stability of having nocturia [4, 10, 45]; and considerations around determining the appropriate time interval for repeated sampling [39].

First, studying nocturia incidence demands repeated, longitudinal assessment of a given population over time. From an epidemiological perspective, longitudinal analyses are preferred over cross-sectional data. Cross-sectional data do not allow distinction between cause and effect, or allow one to understand factors that are associated in terms of exposure and disease. Understanding modifiable risk factors and the pathogenesis of disease becomes easier when the time course is explicit. Having longitudinal assessments implies a greater stability of an investigative team and funding, making such data rarer. Given that the commonly used ICS definition of nocturia was published relatively recently in 2002 [3] – given the long lead-time needed to develop a longitudinal cohort, longitudinal studies on nocturia are rarer still. Several investigators who have published cross-sectional analysis are waiting for longitudinal data to become available. It is highly likely that several new articles regarding nocturia incidence will become available as cohorts are followed.

A second aspect of studying nocturia incidence is consideration as to whether there is a clear and meaningful distinction between "having" nocturia and "not having" nocturia. The ICS definition provides a framework as to what is and what is not nocturia, which includes any episode of waking from sleep at night to void [3]. Literature published subsequently strongly suggests that once one has nocturia twice nightly, the condition more likely is relevant as a quality-of-life concern [40–43]. The use of non-standard case definitions will make the study of incidence and comparisons across studies much more difficult.

A third consideration is whether or not the states of having or not having nocturia are durable or irreversible. Having other certain conditions, such as human immunodeficiency virus (HIV), stroke, prostate cancer or ulcerative colitis, might be considered transformative in comparison. In these examples, incidence is more easily defined with a baseline state of relative health followed by a clear and irreversible state where the condition is present. While nocturia may have remission and incidence and varying presentation over time, cross-sectional data clearly demonstrate that older adults have a much higher prevalence of nocturia than do younger adults. In the absence of a distinct birth-cohort difference, there must be development of nocturia incidence over time.

Fourth, in situations where conditions are not permanent and might come and go, the time frame for sampling becomes important. In conditions with less permanence – examples would include conditions such as influenza, urinary tract infections or delirium – the timing and frequency of questioning become critical. Yet still, one recognises that an incident case might have a period of being afflicted by the condition, usually followed by a return to the state of relative health.

From this state of health, one could remain free of the condition forever, or might return to a state of being afflicted again. In this situation of incidence, remission and the possibility of repeated incidence, the appropriate time frame must be considered. Ideally, there would be some understanding of how long the condition might last so that a sampling time frame that is appropriate could be used. In the example of influenza, there is a defined season roughly between September and March, so individuals are assumed to have returned to relative health in April through August. One can begin to see that an individual could develop influenza in October and a different strain in February. A time frame of sampling on a yearly basis would likely miss such cases.

A final important consideration is that incidence studies require that a population without nocturia must be followed over a specified period of time and again assessed to detect the development of the condition. Many prevalence studies on nocturia have demonstrated, particularly when examining older population cohorts, that the proportion of individuals reporting having zero episodes of nocturia is often the minority of respondents. Considering this framework, one begins to understand some of the problems of studying nocturia incidence.

Published studies of nocturia prevalence greatly outnumber nocturia incidence studies. Prevalence studies may involve representative samples, but often they utilise convenience or clinical samples of participants, and usually employ a single survey or questionnaire. Several studies describing "nocturia incidence" were actually cross-sectional surveys [22, 44]; the *incidence* being described was the higher prevalence of nocturia in the older compared to the younger cohort. Longitudinal studies require identification of a sample with a plan and resources that allows the population to be followed over time. The effort, costs and organisational structure required make longitudinal follow-up much more difficult, yet distinct advantages result.

First, only longitudinal studies can be used to determine incidence. Second, these studies allow distinction between a risk factor (which must come first) and outcome (which must follow), which can allow for a meaningful approach as to how to eliminate or postpone the development of nocturia. Third, incidence data allow one to separate cohort from calendar effects. For example, is the high prevalence of nocturia amongst 80-year olds in 2005 related to risk factors for nocturia for octogenarians, or related to risk factors for those born in 1925?

Few longitudinal studies have examined a cohort recruited from the general population to study the incidence of nocturia [45]. The Medical Epidemiologic and Social Aspects (MESA) study surveyed male and female adults over 60 living in the community in Washtenaw County, Michigan (USA). [46] Participants were seen in their homes in 1983–1984 and three times subsequently. Nocturia was ascertained by ordinal response (0,1,2,3,4,5,6,7,8,9,10 or more) to the question "Generally, how many times do you usually urinate after you have gone to sleep at night" during the baseline and first- and second-year follow-ups. Nocturia was dichotomized as present (2 or more episodes) versus absent (0 or 1 episodes) and incident nocturia was defined by following those with no nocturia at baseline out to year two. Of the 738 individuals with no nocturia at baseline, 34.6% (259) reported having nocturia (2 *or more*) at follow-up, or an incidence rate of 213/1,000 person-years. Of individuals who had two or more episodes at baseline (357), 237 (66.3%) reported one or fewer at follow-up, for a remittance rate of 497/1,000 person years. Amongst risk factors examined, only age was a risk factor for subsequent development of nocturia and only for incidence at 1 year. Contributing to the imprecision of these estimates were that the exact number of days between date at baseline and date at follow-up was not calculated, and that age-specific and gender-specific incidence and remission rates were not determined. [45]

Subsequent work (Tampere Aging Male Urologic Study, TAMUS) within a representative population of men in Pirkanmaa County, Finland, surveyed by postal questionnaire at baseline, 5 and 10 years was stronger in several respects [47]. The nocturia question was from a translation of the DAN-PSS-1 ("how many times do you have to void per night?") with available response categories of 0, 1–2, 3–4 and 5 *or more (times per night)*. Incidence was examined for transitions from *zero* to *one or more* and for *0–2* to *3 or more*. Incidence ratios were also calculated separately for the 50, 60 and 70-year old cohorts. The crude incidence of nocturia for men from *zero* to *one or more* was 75 new cases per 1,000 person-years (95% CI: 66 to 85) during the first 5-year period and 126 (95% CI: 113 to 140) new cases during the second period. Younger cohorts (50 years old) had lower incidence (61 cases/1,000 person-years) than did the two older cohorts (60+ and 70+ year cohort, 91 or 93 new cases/1,000 person-years, respectively). Interestingly, for all age cohorts the rate of incidence during the second 5-year period was higher than during the first: 102, 168 and 167 per person years of follow-up for 50-, 60- and 70-year olds. Given that the several studies have demonstrated that nocturia is likely meaningful once it occurs two or more times [40–43], the incidence of severe nocturia in this study might be more clinically relevant. The incidence of nocturia to three or more times (from 0 or 1–2 times) was less across all age groups (3/1,000 person years for 50–55 year olds, 12/1,000 for 60–65 year olds and 16/1,000 for 70–75 year olds). Interestingly, calendar time yielded a higher prevalence of nocturia (for example, prevalence for 60 year olds was higher at 10-year follow-up than was prevalence for 70-year olds at baseline). Due to the response categories used in questioning, no information is available about incidence of nocturia from ≤ 1 episode to ≥ 2 or more. This makes it difficult to compare data across studies. Also, little insight into nocturia in women can be gained. [47]

In a separate study in Denmark [48, 49], 305 women of child-bearing age were followed after their first pregnancy (278 women responded at 5 years and 242 at 12 years) to examine the incidence (and remittance) of lower urinary tract symptoms. Nocturia, defined here as *voiding twice or more during nighttime*, was highly common during pregnancy, yet was the only urinary symptom tracked that decreased after first childbirth. Of 157 women who had no nocturia during pregnancy, not a single one developed it at 3 months. Of those having no nocturia at 3 month follow-up, 6 of 225 (2.7%) developed two or more episodes of nocturia by 5 years, and 13 developed nocturia at 12 years out of the 220 (5.9%) who had no nocturia at 5 years. Nocturia resolved in 98.6% of women (68/69) who experienced it during pregnancy, by 3 months post-partum. Several physiological factors (reduction in plasma volume, renal night-time solute excretion and decreased functional bladder capacity) which resolved during this time frame likely account for this observation. While remittance of nocturia was tracked to 5 and 12 years, the number of respondents within these categories was very small (1 person and 4 people) as was the proportion having the symptom (1 and 6 persons). [48]

With a well-executed longitudinal study, one may study risk factors associated with the incidence (or remission) of nocturia. An important finding from the TAMUS study related to the incidence of nocturia was its relation with depression (by mental health inventory, MHI-5 instrument) [50]. Depression increased the incidence of nocturia; importantly to know, nocturia did not increase the incidence of depression. Further, for each unit of increment on the short form of the MHI-5 (scale of 5 to 30), the incidence rate ratio of moderate or severe nocturia increased by 10%. The authors concluded that "untreated depressive symptoms may cause nocturia." However, they actually did not assess the use of anti-depressant medication but the use of "any psychiatric medication" which may have effect [50]. Additionally, in the TAMUS study [51], a higher body mass index (BMI) ($\geq$ 30 vs. the comparison group 18.5–24.9) also increased the risk of development of nocturia; 1.6 (95% CI 1.1–2.4) for mild nocturia and 2.3 (95% CI 1.1–4.7) for moderate to severe nocturia. Nocturia at baseline was not associated with increased obesity at follow-up confirming earlier reports of obesity as a risk factor for nocturia [8, 52, 53]. Futhermore, while moderate alcohol usage decreased risk of nocturia incidence versus abstention for moderate to severe nocturia, there was no clear relationship between greater consumption nor was there a statistically significant relationship for the incidence of mild nocturia [51].

Given that there are only a few incidence studies on nocturia, clear and consistent relationships demonstrated consistently across populations and using different methodologies or different definitions do not yet exist. From the available data, it appears that there are fewer risk factors identified for incident nocturia than for prevalent nocturia, that older adults have a higher incidence (and lower remissions) of nocturia than do younger adults, that the incidence of mild nocturia is higher than severe nocturia and that the pronounced remittance of nocturia in the immediate post-partum period is in distinct contrast to the incidence of other LUTS. Also, depression increases nocturia incidence while nocturia is unrelated to the incidence of depression. What remains unclear is the incidence of nocturia in women and how nocturia is affected by the use of nocturia self reports and their inherent instability.

Impact of Nocturia

Bother of Nocturia and Impact on Quality of Life

Urinary storage symptoms, such as nocturia, urgency and increased daytime frequency have been reported to cause more bother than voiding symptoms, such as weak stream or incomplete emptying [54, 55]. Besides intrinsic bother [25, 40, 42, 54, 56], nocturia entails sleep loss, daytime fatigue, missed work, lower perceived health, depression [20, 57, 58] and is associated with impaired quality of life [42, 59].

There is a growing body of evidence regarding the negative effects of disturbed sleep on health, mood, morbidity and ultimately also on mortality [60–62]. Nocturnal micturition is associated with sleep disorders and increased daytime fatigue [57]. It is suggested that bothersomeness of nocturia is primarily related to sleep; however, there is little evidence for this in the literature [63, 64]. In some studies, nocturia was the most important reason for nocturnal awakenings leading possibly to sleep maintenance insomnia [65–67]. On the contrary, in a US sleep-centre study, sleep apnea and other sleep disorders were responsible for the majority of nocturia [68].

Deciding the level of nocturia that constitutes "too often" is a meaningful, practical and theoretical consideration. Bothersome symptoms of patients should not be ignored; alternatively, expected symptoms should not be excessively "medicalised". Does nocturia become abnormal with one or two episodes, or should that number be three or four? Although more frequent nocturia causes more bother, the relationship is not perfectly correlated [22, 25, 29, 40–42, 69–71].

Most studies on the impact of nocturia on health have been inconsistent or non-specific regarding how the degree of nocturia affects bother. In one study, nocturia of "two or more times per night" was associated with lower self-rated physical and mental health [53]. Elsewhere, female patients were shown to seek medical advice about nocturia if they averaged three or more episodes [72]. There is also evidence suggesting that the impact of nocturia may differ by gender. Early use of the International Consultation on Incontinence Modular Questionnaire–Nocturia Quality of Life questionnaire in a mixed gender population suggested that the impact of nocturia was greater for women [41]. By contrast, the effect size of the association for nocturia and major depression may be twice as great in men than in women [73].

The FINNO Study examined the bother and quality of life impact of nocturia by age and sex, and the relationship between nocturia frequency and bother, and nocturia frequency and quality of life [42]. Most respondents reported some bother from nocturia with ≥2 episodes per night, and moderate bother only with ≥3 nocturia episodes (Fig. 5.4). Of the FINNO Study respondents (regardless of nocturia frequency), 4% reported moderate bother from nocturia, while only 1% reported that waking up at night to urinate was a major bother. Overall, among those with any nocturia, approximately one in eight reported moderate or major bother, while both no and small bother was reported by slightly more than 40% of the subjects with nocturia (Fig. 5.4). Generally, degree of bother increased with nocturia frequency [42].

In the FINNO Study, those with two nocturia episodes also reported substantially impaired health-related quality of life compared to those with no nocturia (Fig. 5.5). At least three episodes of nocturia resulted in further impairment of similar magnitude. Using a standardised measure of a clinically important difference in 15D score [74], those reporting a single nocturia episode were not notably different from those reporting none. In both sexes, subjects with ≥3 voids/night reported poorer health-related quality of life (HRQL) than subjects either without nocturia, or with 1–2 voids/night [42].

5 Epidemiology of Nocturia: Evaluation of Prevalence, Incidence... 87

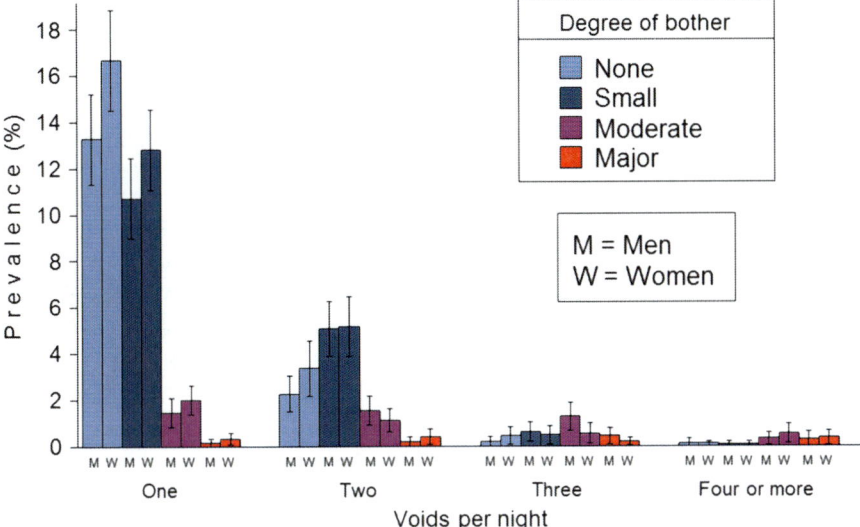

Fig. 5.4 Prevalence of bother by frequency of nocturia (1, 2, 3, or ≥4 voids per night) among men and women in the FINNO Study, Finland, 2003–2004. Age standardisation performed using the age structure of Finland (beginning of 2004). Error bars represent 95% confidence intervals. Modified from [42]

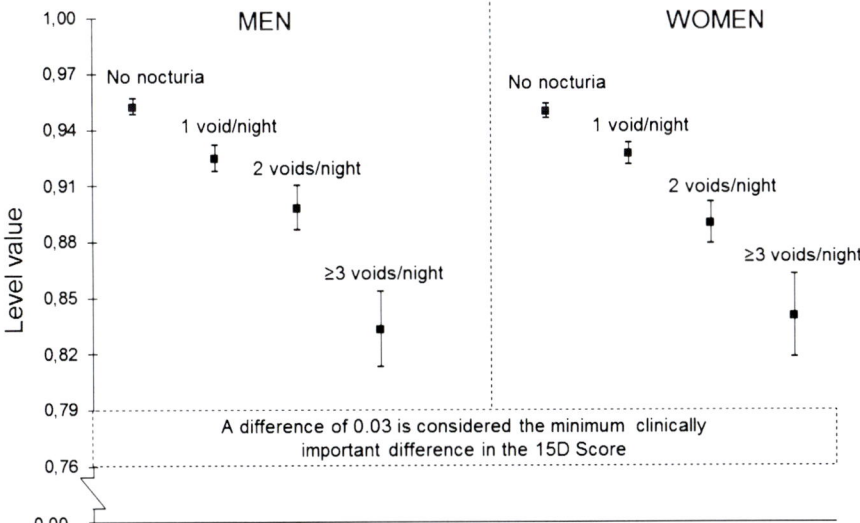

Fig. 5.5 The age-adjusted means for health-related quality of life 15D score [74] by frequency of nocturia in the FINNO Study, Finland, 2003–2004. Age standardisation performed using the age structure of Finland (beginning of 2004). *Error bars* represent 95% confidence intervals. Modified from [11]

Overall, the FINNO Study findings indicated that two episodes of nocturia constitute meaningful nocturia, affecting well-being and perceived health. Most respondents report bother from nocturia only with two or more nightly nocturia episodes, and associate moderate bother only with three or more nocturia episodes. Furthermore, two nightly voids were also associated with a clinically important decrease in health-related quality of life whereas a single episode was not [42]. Hence, the FINNO Study results suggest that one void per night does not identify subjects with interference from nocturia, making it an unsuitable criterion for clinically relevant nocturia [42].

One US study found that scores from OAB-q, an HRQL instrument designed specifically for OAB, differed statistically significantly between subjects with one, two and three episodes of nocturia. However, the clinical importance of these differences remained unclear [25]. Another study among US female urology clinic patients and a Taiwanese community-based study also proposed that clinically significant nocturia (based on bother) is ≥2 voids per night [29, 40]. In another US urogynaecology clinic-based study [71], the mean bother score ≥5 out of 10 was reported only with ≥3 nocturia episodes. In Asian population-based studies and a Viennese health-screening study, nocturia was no problem [29, 70] or not more than "a bit of problem" [22] for most respondents.

In the FINNO Study, men and women generally reported similar overall bother from nocturia [42]. Although older women were less bothered than younger women, no such difference was observed among men. While the prevalence of nocturia increases with age, the prevalence of nocturia in men rises more steeply (Figs. 5.2–5.3). A plausible explanation may be that older women become accustomed reporting less bother from nocturia as they are less likely to develop it as a "new" condition with increasing age. A Viennese health-screening study reported no gender differences in bother from nocturia [22]. A population-based study in Taiwan among adults over 40 years showed that men reported more bother and concern related to nocturia than women [41]. However, a Danish survey of adults aged 60–80 showed that women with ≥3 nocturia episodes were more bothered than men. In less severe nocturia, however, no gender difference was found [66]. The Danish study also showed that nocturia caused more concern in younger age groups.

While more frequent nocturia results in greater bother and poorer HRQL [42], many studies have shown that not all bother from nocturia is explained by the number of nocturia episodes. Nocturia may also be associated with other factors causing impaired HRQL, rather than directly affecting self-rated health [11]. This is supported by the FINNO Study finding of an association of nocturia with almost all dimensions of HRQL. There were prominent effects within not only closely related domains including eliminating and sexual activity, but also ostensibly unrelated areas including moving, seeing and hearing [42]. Furthermore, co-morbidities were strongly associated with impaired HRQL, and also with nocturia, indicating confounding. Treatment to reduce episodes of nocturia may therefore not relieve all impairment among subjects with nocturia [11]. Indeed, nocturia may also be considered as a typical *geriatric syndrome* (i.e., one symptom or a complex of symptoms with high prevalence in old age, resulting from multiple diseases and multiple risk factors) [75].

Impact of Nocturia on Falls, Fractures and Mortality

Falls are the greatest single risk factor for fractures in elderly people [76]. Nocturia has been associated with an increased risk of both falls and fractures [77–83]. Furthermore, two earlier [84, 85] and two recent [30, 83] studies have reported a link between nocturia and mortality. In a longitudinal community-based study among Japanese elderly [83], nocturia (defined as at least two voids/night) was associated with doubled risk of both fractures and mortality. Parallel mortality effects were also found in a recent population-based US study. However, effect sizes were smaller: 49% increased mortality risk for men and 32% for women (nocturia definition of at least two voids/night was used also here) [30]. Whether falls, fractures and increased mortality are due to nocturnal visits to the lavatory, daytime fatigue secondary to nocturia, or other co-morbidities, is not clear. It is also possible that nocturia does not directly cause falls and increased mortality risk but is associated with factors causing them – being an indicator of frailty [11]. There is no randomised controlled trial assessing the impact of nocturia treatment in prevention of falls, fractures and increased mortality risk.

Risk Factors (See Also Chap. 2)

The causes and risk factors of nocturia are not well understood [4, 11]. Current understanding of nocturia (Table 5.1) is based mainly on *expert opinions* rather than *scientific evidence* [86, 87]. Our aim in this section is to summarise the most important potential risk factors of nocturia identified in the current literature. The following (in alphabetical order) are the main risk factors identified as being associated with nocturia.

Conditions

Benign Prostatic Hyperplasia. Many individuals with nocturia, particularly elderly men, have other LUTS (such as urinary frequency, weak stream, urgency) and these symptoms are most often attributed to BPH/benign prostatic enlargement (BPE)/benign prostatic obstruction (BPO) in men [2]. In the population-based FINNO Study [88], BPH had the second highest population-attributable fraction of nocturia for men (after OAB). However, the odds ratio of BPH for nocturia was 2.1 (95% CI 1.2–3.7), while many other conditions had clearly higher odds ratios in the multivariate analysis, though differences (between conditions) were mainly statistically non-significant [88]. Overall, half of the subjects with physician-diagnosed BPH reported at least two voids per night – only yet a third of the men with nocturia reported BPH (Fig. 5.6). Overall, LUTS suggestive of BPH/BPO constitute a

Table 5.1 Factors proposed as involved in etiology of nocturia

Urological conditions (in alphabetical order)		
Bladder outlet obstruction	Detrusor overactivity	Painful bladder syndrome
Bladder hypersensitivity	Interstitial cystitis	Pelvic floor laxity (cystocele, uterine prolapse, etc)
Calculi of bladder or ureter	Learned voiding dysfunction	
Bladder, prostate or urethra cancer	Neurogenic bladder	Sensory urgency
Decreased bladder capacity	Overactive bladder (syndrome)	Urine tract infection
Non-urological conditions (in alphabetical order)		
Aging	Excessive fluid intake	Peripheral edema
Anxiety	Hypercalcemia	Pharmacological agents such as: alcohol, β-blockers, caffeine, calcium-channel blockers, diuretics, lithium, selective serotonine reuptake inhibitors, theophylline, etc
Autonomic dysfunction	Hypoalbuminemia	
Chronic kidney disease	Hypokalemia	
Chronic obstructive lung disease	Insomnia	
Chronic pain	Multiple sclerosis	
Congestive heart failure	Nephrosis	
Defect in secretion or action of antidiuretic hormone	Neurodegenerative conditions (Parkinsonism or Alzheimer's)	Periodic limb movement disorder
		Pruritus
Depression	Nocturnal polyuria	Restless legs syndrome
Diabetes mellitus/insipidus	Nocturnal epileptic seizures	Sleep apnea
Dyspnea	Oestrogen deficiency	Venous insufficiency

Modified from [11, 110, 174–178]

well-recognised risk factor for nocturia [34, 89]. However, the impact of BPH may be overestimated (nocturic men probably are more likely to be BPH diagnosed than men without nocturia, and women do not have less nocturia despite not having prostates). In Japanese studies, nocturia was the least specific LUTS associated with BPO and treatment to relieve BPO had less effect on nocturia than on other symptoms [90, 91]. Rate of nocturia improvement was 13.9% in tamsulosin group and 19.6% in the transurethral resection of the prostate (TURP) group [91]. Other six LUTS assessed were each improved in 18.2–28.5% of patients in the tamsulosin and in 37.0–63.0% of patients in the TURP group respectively. Furthermore, in a secondary analysis of the Veterans Affairs study on participants with LUTS/BPH, those receiving doxazosin had very modest (though statistically significant) reductions in nocturia, while finasteride had an effect indistinguishable from placebo [92]. Concurring these findings, already in the 1970s and 1980s, nocturia had been reported as one of the most (if not the single most) persistent LUTS following prostate surgery [93, 94].

Depression. In a Swedish population-based study [73], subjects with major depression (assessed by the Major Depression Inventory [95]) reported substantially more nocturia than those without. The association was especially strong among men

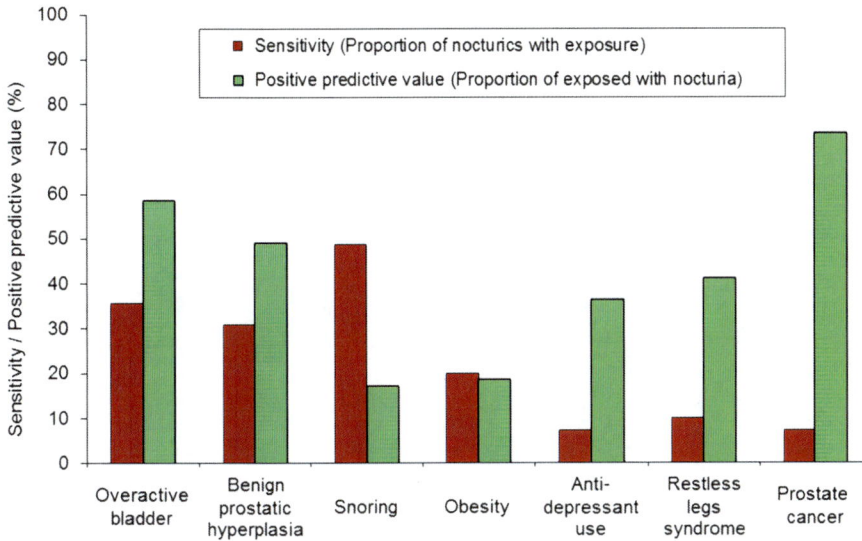

Fig. 5.6 Sensitivity and positive predictive value for factors associated with nocturia among *men* in the population-based FINNO Study, Finland, 2003–2004. BPH refers to benign prostatic hyperplasia, AD use to antidepressant use, and RLS to restless legs syndrome. Obesity was defined as body mass index of 30 kg/m^2 or more. Modified from [88] (which is an Open Access article distributed under the terms of the Creative Commons Attribution Non-Commercial License which permits unrestricted non-commercial use, distribution and reproduction in any medium, provided the original work is properly cited)

(OR 6.5, 95% CI 2.6–15.6 for men, and OR 2.8, 95% CI 1.3–6.3 for women, adjusted for age and somatic health). However, in a subsequent analysis from the same database [96], the authors reported that both major depression (OR 4.6, 95% CI 2.8–7.5) and taking an SSRI (OR 2.2; 95% CI 1.1–4.5) were associated with increased prevalence of nocturia (gender was deleted by the logistic regression model). In the TAMUS cohort study (conducted among men aged 50 or more), those with depressive symptoms at study entry were at 2.8 times higher risk (95% CI 1.5–5.2) for moderate or severe nocturia (defined as at least three voids/night) than those without depressive symptoms, but nocturia had no effect on depressive symptoms during 5-year follow-up. In the FINNO Study [88], nocturia was associated with anti-depressant use only in men (OR 3.2, 95% CI 1.3–7.7). Depression itself was not associated with nocturia after adjustment for other factors despite associations in the age-adjusted analyses (OR 2.8, 95% CI: 1.6, 5.0 for men; and OR 2.0, 95% CI: 1.2, 3.3 for women).

Hypertension and Coronary Disease. It has been proposed that nocturnal polyuria and essential hypertension are manifestations of the same pathophysiological process [97]. However, the connection between nocturia and hypertension is not clear. In a Japanese health screening study (OR 1.6, 95% CI 1.5–1.9) [26] and in a US population-based study among elderly (OR 1.5, 95% CI 1.2–1.9) [45], hypertension

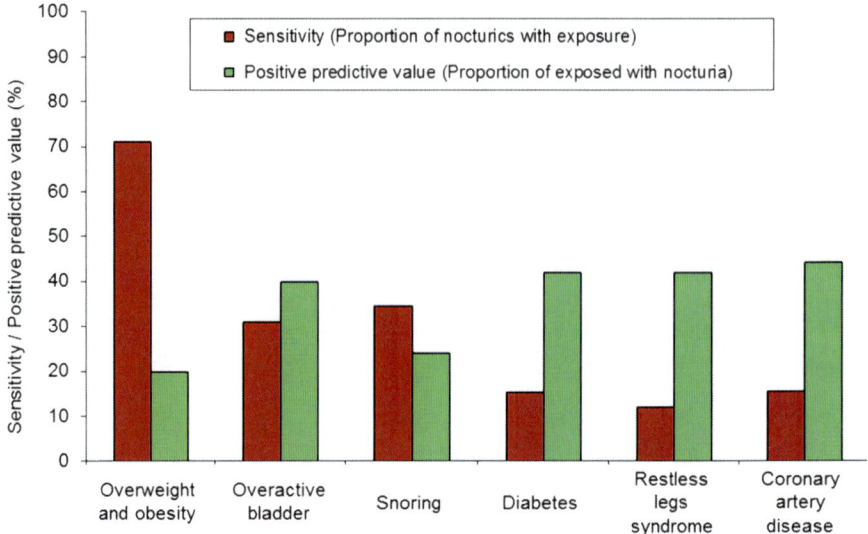

Fig. 5.7 Sensitivity and positive predictive value for factors associated with nocturia among *women* in the population-based FINNO Study, Finland, 2003–2004. RLS refers to restless legs syndrome and CAD to coronary artery disease. Overweight was defined as body mass index of 25–30 kg/m^2 and obesity as 30 kg/m^2 or more. Modified from [88] (which is an Open Access article distributed under the terms of the Creative Commons Attribution Non-Commercial License which permits unrestricted non-commercial use, distribution and reproduction in any medium, provided the original work is properly cited)

was associated with nocturia. However, in studies conducted in the Netherlands, Sweden and Finland [24, 34, 88], nocturnal polyuria or nocturia were not associated with hypertension. Appropriate research methodology is of particular importance when assessing the impact of hypertension on nocturia: for example, treatment of hypertension with calcium-channel blockers and poorly timed versus "properly" timed diuretics may cause [2, 98] or alleviate nocturia [99].

Cardiac disease, coronary disease and congestive heart failure have been proposed as causal or risk factors for nocturia in most reviews (Table 5.1). Earlier studies conducted mainly among men [24, 26, 34] did not find relationships between cardiac disease and nocturia. In all these studies [24, 26, 34], an association between cardiac symptoms/disease and nocturia was found in the preliminary analyses before multivariate models. However, in several more recent studies, [53, 85, 88, 100] coronary disease has been shown to be associated with nocturia. In the Boston Area Community Health Survey [53], the association of nocturia with cardiac disease persisted in the multivariate model (OR 1.4, 95% CI 1.0–1.7). In the FINNO Study, coronary artery disease was associated with nocturia in the age-adjusted analyses in both sexes, but after adjustment for other factors the association persisted only for women (OR 3.1, 95% CI 1.5–6.6) [88]. Almost half of the women with coronary artery disease reported at least two voids/night while every sixth woman with nocturia reported coronary artery disease (Fig. 5.7).

Neurological Diseases. Several neurological conditions are potentially causal factors for OAB-type of symptoms [101–103]. Less is known about the impact of neurological diseases on nocturia. Most patients with multiple sclerosis (approximately 75%) have bladder dysfunction leading to urinary storage symptoms [101, 104], and potentially to nocturia. In Swedish and Dutch studies on elderly people, nocturia was associated with stroke (OR 2.0, 95% CI 1.1–3.6) and cerebrovascular disease (OR 1.8, 1.2–2.7), respectively [100, 105]. Sleeping problems and nocturia are common among Parkinson's patients [106]. In a study among Parkinson's patients, severity of disease was also associated with increased nocturia (mean of nocturia episodes was 1.8 in the mild, and 2.9 in the severe Parkinson groups) [107].

Nocturia was found to be related to restless legs syndrome in the FINNO Study [88]. Subjects of both sexes with restless legs syndrome (compared to those without) had almost triple the risk of having nocturia (men: OR 2.9, 95% CI 1.3–6.5; women: OR 2.9, 95% CI 1.4–5.8). While almost half of those with restless legs syndrome had nocturia, only one out of eight with nocturia had restless legs syndrome. To the best of our knowledge, other studies have not examined this link. Increased risk of nocturia in patients with restless legs syndrome may relate to disturbed sleep [108]. Moreover, restless legs syndrome patients use medications such as anti-depressants, gastrointestinal medications and asthma/allergy drugs more frequently than subjects free of them [109].

Nocturnal Polyuria. According to the ICS [110], nocturnal polyuria is present when an increased proportion of the 24-h output occurs at night. However, there is a dire lack of studies to provide reference values. In the population-based Krimpen study (see also Chap. 4), nocturia was strongly associated with nocturnal polyuria [34]. However, it was difficult to separate men with and without increased voiding frequency on the basis of nocturnal urine production [34, 111]. Among these men, nocturnal urine production was slightly more than 60 ml/h. The authors suggested that nocturnal urine production exceeding 90 ml/h is abnormal. However, the authors concluded that "nocturnal urine production as an explanatory variable for nocturnal voiding frequency is of little value." [111] Overall, the fundamental pathogenesis of nocturnal polyuria is difficult to assess. Congestive heart failure, "third spacing" (venous insufficiency, nephrosis) or late-night diuretic administration are potential underlying causes. There is increasing recent evidence on the impact of edema on nocturia and nocturnal polyuria. Using bioelectric impedance analysis, Japanese researchers investigated the relation between nocturnal polyuria and the variation of body fluid distribution during the daytime [112]. Nocturnal urine volume significantly correlated with the difference in fluid volume in the legs ($r=0.53$, $p=0.002$) and extracellular fluid volume ($r=0.38$, $p=0.02$) between the morning and evening volumes. These findings were indirectly supported by the results of a non-randomised study where the number of nocturia episodes decreased significantly ($p<0.001$) from 3.3 to 1.9 after 8 weeks of walking exercise in Japanese elderly men [113]. Possible other pathways to nocturnal polyuria also include diminished renal concentrating capacity, diminished sodium conserving ability, loss of the circadian rhythm of antidiuretic hormone secretion, decreased secretion of renin-angiotensin-aldosterone, and increased secretion of atrial natriuretic hormone (e.g., due to obstructive sleep apnea) leading to increased night-time urine production [114–116]. The pathophysiology of nocturnal polyuria merits further studies.

Obesity and Diabetes. Several studies have shown the relation of overweight/obesity and nocturia. In a Swedish population-based study among middle-aged women, obesity (but not overweight) was associated with nocturia (BMI ≥30: OR 3.5, 95% CI 2.6–4.7; BMI <20 as reference) [52]. In the FINNO Study [8, 88], overweight/obesity had the greatest impact on nocturia at population level among women. Obesity was associated with more than doubled risk of nocturia among both sexes after multivariate analyses (OR 2.1, 95% CI 1.2–3.6 for men, and OR 2.2 95% CI 1.3–3.7 for women). Confirmatory findings have been reported in recent cross-sectional studies [53, 117, 118] as well as in the TAMUS cohort study (conducted among men aged 50 or more) [51], where obese men were at higher risk for both mild nocturia (RR 1.6, 95%CI 1.1–2.4) and especially for moderate or severe nocturia (RR 2.3, 95%CI 1.1–4.7) compared with normal-weight men. The frequency of nocturia at baseline did not increase the incidence of obesity at follow-up [51]. Potentially, preventing obesity may decrease nocturia, though establishing causality would ideally require an intervention study. Weight loss has been already shown to decrease urinary incontinence substantially among overweight and obese women [119].

An association between diabetes and nocturia has been reported in most [26, 53, 88, 89, 100, 105, 118, 120–122], but not all reports [24, 34, 45]. In the Boston Area Community Health Survey [53] and in a Danish study at ages 60–80 years [118], nocturia was associated with diabetes (OR 1.7, 95% CI 1.2–2.3 in the Boston and OR 2.0, 95% CI 1.3–3.0 in the Danish study). In both surveys [53, 118], adjustment for sex was used, but it was not clear whether there were gender differences in risk factors. In the FINNO Study [88], diabetes was associated with nocturia in the age-adjusted analyses in both sexes, but after adjustment for other factors the association persisted only for women (OR 2.7, 95% CI 1.4–5.2).

Overactive Bladder and Detrusor Overactivity. According to the ICS, OAB is a symptom-defined condition characterised by urinary urgency, with or without urgency incontinence, usually with increased daytime frequency and nocturia [110, 123]. It is commonly proposed that urinary urgency is the primary driver of all symptoms of the OAB constellation including increased nocturia [124]. Recent evidence using nocturnal cystometrography has indeed confirmed a temporal relationship between nocturnal detrusor overactivity and nocturic voids is some patients [125]. In a British study among women aged 40 or more [126], self-reported nocturia predicted urodynamically confirmed detrusor overactivity (OR 1.9, 95% CI 1.1–3.3, OR 2.0, 95% CI 1.1–3.8, and OR 3.1 95% CI 1.4–6.6 for women with one, two and three or more void(s) per night, respectively). Further, urinary urgency was a clear risk factor for nocturia in the FINNO Study (OR 7.4, 95% CI 4.5–12 for men, and OR 4.9, 95% CI 3.2–7.7 for women) [88]. However, while half of the subjects with urgency also reported at least two voids per night, only one in three with nocturia reported urgency [127] (Fig. 5.8). Despite these findings, the treatment of nocturia with bladder relaxants (antimuscarinics) is often unsuccessful [128].

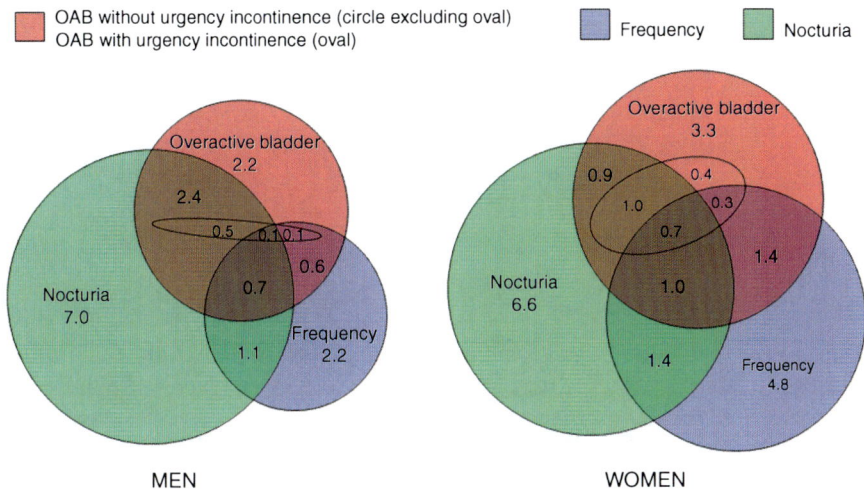

Fig. 5.8 Age-standardised prevalence of nocturia, overactive bladder (with or without urgency incontinence) and urinary frequency among people aged 18–79 years in the population-based FINNO Study, Finland, 2003–2004. The *red circle* represents subjects with overactive bladder without urgency incontinence excluding the area of the *red oval* representing subjects with overactive bladder with urgency incontinence. The *blue circle* represents subjects with urinary frequency (defined as more than eight voids/day) and the *green circle* nocturia (defined as more at least two voids/night). Age standardisation performed using the age structure of Finland (beginning of 2004). Modified from [127] (which is an Open Access article distributed under the terms of the Creative Commons Attribution Non-Commercial License which permits unrestricted non-commercial use, distribution and reproduction in any medium, provided the original work is properly cited)

Prostate Cancer. Many men with LUTS express a fear of prostate cancer [129] and many physicians use prostate-specific antigen for ruling out prostate cancer as a part of initial evaluation of male patients with LUTS. This is in accordance with many guidelines such as the current AUA BPH guideline which recommends PSA screening in "patients with at least a 10-year life expectancy for whom knowledge of the presence of prostate cancer would change management, or patients [in] whom the PSA measurement may change the management of voiding symptoms" [130]. However, not much is known whether LUTS really are suggestive of prostate cancer [131], and even less about whether nocturia predicts prostate cancer or vice versa. In the large population-based HUNT-2 study, severity of LUTS was positively associated with the subsequent diagnosis of localised prostate cancer but authors found no evidence for a positive association with advanced or fatal disease. These findings are in line with the FINNO Study results: nocturia was associated with physician-diagnosed prostate cancer [88]. More than 70% of men with physician-diagnosed prostate cancer reported at least two voids/night, while 7% of men with nocturia reported prostate cancer. However, it remains unclear whether the subjects with nocturia are more vulnerable to be diagnosed (due to use of prostate-specific antigen among men with LUTS), whether prostate cancer really causes nocturia, or whether nocturia is a side-effect of various prostate cancer treatments [42, 132]. More SUI and less obstructive symptoms have been reported after radical prostatectomy whereas impact on nocturia has been neutral or negative (i.e., increased nocturia) [133–135]. The lack of association of advanced prostate cancer and LUTS severity [136] contradicts the hypothesis that prostate cancer causes LUTS.

Lifestyle

Coffee and Alcohol. Both coffee and alcohol are diuretic liquids with the potential to increase urine volumes. Treatment guidelines usually recommend decreasing (bedtime) fluid intake, especially coffee and alcohol (Table 5.1). However, most studies have not found any relation between nocturia and coffee/caffeine [20, 51, 52, 88, 137] or alcohol [22, 26, 45, 88, 118, 138]. In some studies, moderate alcohol consumers had a lower prevalence of nocturia than abstainers [51, 100, 139]. Although there could theoretically be several biological factors behind this association, a *systematic misclassification error* (including people who decrease or finish drinking due to ill health to abstainer category) [140, 141] or *residual confounding* (moderate drinkers have many favouring social and lifestyle factors which are not likely not due to alcohol consumption itself) [142, 143] could also explain this.

Smoking. Most studies have not found an association for nocturia with smoking [20, 51, 85, 88, 118, 137, 138]. Some conflicting results have also been reported: in a Swedish study [52], smoking was associated with increased nocturia, whereas in Austrian [22] and Japanese [26] studies, smoking was associated with decreased nocturia. In the population-based Krimpen study [111], smoking reinforced the circadian rhythm in favour of daytime urine production.

Physical Activity. Few studies have assessed the impact of physical activity on nocturia, and in those available, it is not always clear if results are adequately adjusted for BMI and other co-morbidities associated with reduced activity. In the analysis of an Austrian health-screening study [22], no relation was found between physical activity and nocturia, whereas in other studies physical activity appears to be protective against LUTS in men with BPH [144–146], and against nocturia specifically in women [52]. Given that exercise programmes appear to improve nocturia [147], these effects deserve to be further explored.

Race/Ethnicity and Socioeconomic Status

Although the impact of socioeconomic status on nocturia is poorly studied, the ethnic variation in nocturia has been extensively explored for US male populations in recent years. However, relatively little research has focussed on these associations in either women or populations in other countries. Within the US, it is consistently noted that black males are approximately twice as likely to report nocturia as other ethnic groups [148–150]. This effect persisted (although attenuated [148, 149]) after adjusting for co-morbidities and socioeconomic status. Similar effects were reported for women participating in the Boston Area Community Health Survey [53] and the Penn Ovarian study [151], with black women being almost twice as likely to report nocturia after adjustment. In addition to these population-based studies, reports from secondary care populations [152, 153] have also suggested that care-seeking black women more commonly report nocturia. However, conflicting results were found in a Kaiser Permanente study [43]. Little is known about the relationship between ethnicity and nocturia outside the United States. In small studies in Taiwan [154, 155] and Scotland [156], association of nocturia and ethnicity have been found. In the Scottish study, the prevalence of nocturnal polyuria was significantly higher in 200 Caucasian men compared to 93 Asian men. Overall, the underlying mechanisms for the association of nocturia with race/ethnicity remain unknown.

In the previous studies, some of the probable risk factors of nocturia (such as sleep apnea) remained unmeasured. This may have explained the found associations at least partly.

Reproductive Factors in Women

Few studies published so far on the relation of nocturia with reproductive and gynaecological factors have focussed on female reproductive factors including pregnancy, parity, menopause, menopausal hormone therapy and hysterectomy, [157] – and even less attention has been given to the relationship of nocturia with delivery mode, episiotomy and multiple gestations [158].

Gravidity/Pregnancy, Parity and Post-partum Period. Nocturia is a common symptom during pregnancy [48, 159, 160]. In a British study, more than 60% of pregnant women (mean age 24, range 19–40 years) reported three or more nocturic voids per week, with highest prevalence of nocturia in the third trimester [160]. Similar results were found in a recent Indian study where authors assessed current LUTS and LUTS before pregnancy, retrospectively (mean age of women was 26.5 years, range: 18–39). Among these pregnant women, nocturia (defined as more than one void per week) was reported by 58.6% of those in the first, 71.9% in the second and 77.0% in the third trimester. Of these women, 50.6% reported that they had nocturia before pregnancy. In the FINNO Study [161], parous women reported more nocturia than nulliparous women (OR [per child; nulliparous as reference] 1.13, 95% CI 1.0–1.3 in the multivariate analyses), which contradicts earlier reports of no association between parity and nocturia [162, 163]. However, earlier studies included only perimenopausal women [162, 163]. The association of nocturia with parity has been suggested to be more likely due to pregnancy itself than physical damage to the urinary tract during delivery [157]. This notion is in concordance with the FINNO Study finding of no difference in nocturia between primi- and multiparous women [161]. Reports on the association between delivery mode and nocturia are unavailable. In addition to parity, the post-partum period was associated with increased nocturia (but not with urgency) in the FINNO Study [161]. During the post-partum period, increased nocturnal voiding may be secondary to increased number of awakenings and insomnia. Most awakenings are for baby care; however, maternal depressed mood could also play a role [164].

Menopause and Hormone Therapy. In the FINNO Study, the post-menopausal period was associated with increased nocturia (OR 2.3, 95 % CI 1.2–4.4; compared to pre-menopausal women) [161], consistent with a Danish population-based study on 40 to 60 year-old women (OR 2.4, 95% CI 1.1–5.2) [162]. Two other studies have also reported increased nocturia in the post-menopausal period [163, 165], whereas another attributed this to ageing rather than menopausal transition [166]. The reason for possible association of menopause and nocturia is not straightforward. Menopause is often associated with sleep disturbances for other reasons including hot flashes, mood disorders and increased sleep-disordered breathing [164]; therefore, the association with nocturia may be secondary in many cases. There are few studies evaluating the effect of menopausal hormone therapy (MHT) on nocturia. In the FINNO Study, there was increased nocturia among women with MHT (compared to pre-menopausal women; OR, 1.8), but the finding was statistically insignificant [161]. In a Swedish population-based study [163], increasing nocturia was associated with MHT but the association did not remain significant in the multivariate analysis. In a small randomised trial [167], those with MHT did not report less (or more) nocturia than those with placebo. This finding was recently confirmed in a randomised trial assessing the effect of vaginal estradiol on urinary storage symptoms after sling surgery [168]. In this Greek study, there was no improvement in nocturia rates with the vaginal estradiol compared to placebo [168].

Pelvic Surgery: Hysterectomy and Stress Urinary Incontinence Operations. Results are inconsistent regarding hysterectomy and nocturia, with hysterectomy variously being associated with decreased [169–171] or increased prevalence of nocturia [162], or not associated with nocturia at all [172, 173]. Many of the differences are probably due to differences in study populations and methods (many studies are limited by inadequate control of potential confounders) [11]. In the FINNO Study, hysterectomised women (pre-menopausal status as a reference) had an OR of 1.8 (95% CI 0.9–3.6) for nocturia, with borderline statistical significance whereas surgery for stress urinary incontinence was not associated with nocturia (OR 0.9, 95% 0.4–2.5) despite relation of urgency with stress incontinence surgery (OR 2.5, 95% CI 1.0–6.1) [161]. However, statistical power was limited regarding analyses on stress incontinence surgery in this study.

Conclusions

Nocturia is one of the – if not the – most common lower urinary tract symptoms. The prevalence of nocturia increases strongly with age: most elderly people report at least one void per night. The prevalence of nocturia is higher among young women than young men, but because the incidence is greater in men, it becomes more common in men in old age. In general, older adults have a higher incidence (and lower remissions) of nocturia than do younger adults, and the incidence of mild nocturia is higher than severe nocturia. Two episodes of nocturia constitute meaningful nocturia, affecting quality of life and perceived health, while a single episode does not. Three or more voids have a moderate effect on well-being. Nocturia may also be associated with an increased risk of falls, fractures and mortality. However, whether this would be due to nocturnal visits to the lavatory, daytime fatigue secondary to nocturia, or other co-morbidities is unclear. It is possible that nocturia is an indicator of overall frailty, rather than a direct cause. There are numerous risk factors for nocturia, including benign prostatic hyperplasia, overactive bladder, obesity, sleep apnea, parity, post-partum and post-menopausal periods. These risk factors include diseases of the lower urinary tract, but also a range of systemic co-morbidities. However, most of the risk factors have been identified for prevalent (and very few for incident) nocturia. Overall, many studies have demonstrated a multi-factorial etiology for nocturia. Because the prevalence of nocturia strongly increases with age, the number of people affected by it will likely increase with shifting of the population structures towards older age groups globally.

References

1. Barker JC, Mitteness LS. Nocturia in the elderly. Gerontologist. 1988;28(1):99–104.
2. Weiss JP, Blaivas JG. Nocturia. J Urol. 2000;163(1):5–12.
3. van Kerrebroeck P, Abrams P, Chaikin D, et al. The standardisation of terminology in nocturia: report from the Standardisation Sub-committee of the International Continence Society. Neurourol Urodyn. 2002;21(2):179–83.
4. Hunskaar S. Epidemiology of nocturia. BJU Int. 2005;96 Suppl 1:4–7.
5. Haylen BT, de Ridder D, Freeman RM, et al. An International Urogynecological Association (IUGA)/International Continence Society (ICS) joint report on the terminology for female pelvic floor dysfunction. Neurourol Urodyn. 2010;29(1):4–20.
6. Weber AM, Abrams P, Brubaker L, et al. The standardization of terminology for researchers in female pelvic floor disorders. Int Urogynecol J Pelvic Floor Dysfunct. 2001;12(3): 178–86.
7. Weiss JP, Wein AJ, van Kerrebroeck P, et al. Nocturia: new directions ICI-RS Think Tank 2010. Neurourol Urodyn. 2011;30(5):700–3.
8. Tikkinen KA, Tammela TL, Huhtala H, Auvinen A. Is nocturia equally common among men and women? A population based study in Finland. J Urol. 2006;175(2):596–600.
9. Bosch JL, Weiss JP. The prevalence and causes of nocturia. J Urol. 2010;184(2):440–6.
10. Moller LA, Lose G, Jorgensen T. Incidence and remission rates of lower urinary tract symptoms at one year in women aged 40–60: longitudinal study. BMJ. 2000;320(7247): 1429–32.
11. Tikkinen KAO. Epidemiology of nocturia – results from the FINNO Study [dissertation]. Tampere: Tampere University Press. http://acta.uta.fi/pdf/978-951-44-8020-1.pdf (2010) Accessed 2 Feb 2011.
12. Britton JP, Dowell AC, Whelan P. Prevalence of urinary symptoms in men aged over 60. Br J Urol. 1990;66(2):175–6.
13. Garraway WM, Collins GN, Lee RJ. High prevalence of benign prostatic hypertrophy in the community. Lancet. 1991;338(8765):469–71.

14. Chute CG, Panser LA, Girman CJ, et al. The prevalence of prostatism: a population-based survey of urinary symptoms. J Urol. 1993;150(1):85–9.
15. Sagnier PP, MacFarlane G, Richard F, Botto H, Teillac P, Boyle P. Results of an epidemiological survey using a modified American Urological Association symptom index for benign prostatic hyperplasia in France. J Urol. 1994;151(5):1266–70.
16. Homma Y, Imajo C, Takahashi S, Kawabe K, Aso Y. Urinary symptoms and urodynamics in a normal elderly population. Scand J Urol Nephrol Suppl. 1994;157:27–30.
17. Malmsten UG, Milsom I, Molander U, Norlen LJ. Urinary incontinence and lower urinary tract symptoms: an epidemiological study of men aged 45 to 99 years. J Urol. 1997;158(5):1733–7.
18. Sommer P, Nielsen KK, Bauer T, et al. Voiding patterns in men evaluated by a questionnaire survey. Br J Urol. 1990;65(2):155–60.
19. Brieger GM, Yip SK, Hin LY, Chung TK. The prevalence of urinary dysfunction in Hong Kong Chinese women. Obstet Gynecol. 1996;88(6):1041–4.
20. Samuelsson E, Victor A, Tibblin G. A population study of urinary incontinence and nocturia among women aged 20–59 years. Prevalence, well-being and wish for treatment. Acta Obstet Gynecol Scand. 1997;76(1):74–80.
21. Pinnock C, Marshall VR. Troublesome lower urinary tract symptoms in the community: a prevalence study. Med J Aust. 1997;167(2):72–5.
22. Schatzl G, Temml C, Schmidbauer J, Dolezal B, Haidinger G, Madersbacher S. Cross-sectional study of nocturia in both sexes: analysis of a voluntary health screening project. Urology. 2000;56(1):71–5.
23. van Dijk L, Kooij DG, Schellevis FG. Nocturia in the Dutch adult population. BJU Int. 2002;90(7):644–8.
24. Rembratt A, Norgaard JP, Andersson KE. Nocturia and associated morbidity in a community-dwelling elderly population. BJU Int. 2003;92(7):726–30.
25. Coyne KS, Zhou Z, Bhattacharyya SK, Thompson CL, Dhawan R, Versi E. The prevalence of nocturia and its effect on health-related quality of life and sleep in a community sample in the USA. BJU Int. 2003;92(9):948–54.
26. Yoshimura K, Terada N, Matsui Y, Terai A, Kinukawa N, Arai Y. Prevalence of and risk factors for nocturia: analysis of a health screening program. Int J Urol. 2004;11(5):282–7.
27. Irwin DE, Milsom I, Hunskaar S, et al. Population-based survey of urinary incontinence, overactive bladder, and other lower urinary tract symptoms in five countries: results of the EPIC study. Eur Urol. 2006;50(6):1306–15.
28. Herschorn S, Gajewski J, Schulz J, Corcos J. A population-based study of urinary symptoms and incontinence: the Canadian Urinary Bladder Survey. BJU Int. 2008;101(1):52–8.
29. Choo MS, Ku JH, Park CH, et al. Prevalence of nocturia in a Korean population aged 40 to 89 years. Neurourol Urodyn. 2008;27(1):60–4.
30. Kupelian V, Fitzgerald MP, Kaplan SA, Norgaard JP, Chiu GR, Rosen RC. Association of nocturia and mortality: results from the Third National Health and Nutrition Examination Survey. J Urol. 2011;185(2):571–7.
31. McGrother CW, Donaldson MM, Shaw C, et al. Storage symptoms of the bladder: prevalence, incidence and need for services in the UK. BJU Int. 2004;93(6):763–9.
32. Parsons M, Tissot W, Cardozo L, et al. Normative bladder diary measurements: night versus day. Neurourol Urodyn. 2007;26(4):465–73.
33. Muscatello DJ, Rissel C, Szonyi G. Urinary symptoms and incontinence in an urban community: prevalence and associated factors in older men and women. Intern Med J. 2001;31(3):151–60.
34. Blanker MH, Bohnen AM, Groeneveld FP, Bernsen RM, Prins A, Ruud Bosch JL. Normal voiding patterns and determinants of increased diurnal and nocturnal voiding frequency in elderly men. J Urol. 2000;164(4):1201–5.
35. Jaffe JS, Ginsberg PC, Silverberg DM, Harkaway RC. The need for voiding diaries in the evaluation of men with nocturia. J Am Osteopath Assoc. 2002;102(5):261–5.

36. Yoshimura K, Terai A. Fluctuation of night time frequency in patients with symptomatic nocturia. Int J Urol. 2005;12(5):469–73.
37. Stav K, Dwyer PL, Rosamilia A. Women overestimate daytime urinary frequency: the importance of the bladder diary. J Urol. 2009;181(5):2176–80.
38. Chancellor MB. What happened when I took OAB drugs? Neurourol Urodyn. 2007;26(7):1057.
39. Yoshimura K, Kamoto T, Tsukamoto T, Oshiro K, Kinukawa N, Ogawa O. Seasonal alterations in nocturia and other storage symptoms in three Japanese communities. Urology. 2007;69(5):864–70.
40. Fiske J, Scarpero HM, Xue X, Nitti VW. Degree of bother caused by nocturia in women. Neurourol Urodyn. 2004;23(2):130–3.
41. Yu HJ, Chen FY, Huang PC, Chen TH, Chie WC, Liu CY. Impact of nocturia on symptom-specific quality of life among community-dwelling adults aged 40 years and older. Urology. 2006;67(4):713–8.
42. Tikkinen KA, Johnson 2nd TM, Tammela TL, et al. Nocturia frequency, bother, and quality of life: how often is too often? A population-based study in Finland. Eur Urol. 2010;57(3):488–96.
43. Lukacz ES, Whitcomb EL, Lawrence JM, Nager CW, Luber KM. Urinary frequency in community-dwelling women: what is normal? Am J Obstet Gynecol. 2009;200(5):552.e1–7.
44. Zhang X, Zhang J, Chen J, et al. Prevalence and risk factors of nocturia and nocturia-related quality of life in the Chinese population. Urol Int. 2011;86(2):173–8.
45. Johnson 2nd TM, Sattin RW, Parmelee P, Fultz NH, Ouslander JG. Evaluating potentially modifiable risk factors for prevalent and incident nocturia in older adults. J Am Geriatr Soc. 2005;53(6):1011–6.
46. Herzog AR, Fultz NH. Prevalence and incidence of urinary incontinence in community-dwelling populations. J Am Geriatr Soc. 1990;38(3):273–81.
47. Häkkinen JT, Hakama M, Shiri R, Auvinen A, Tammela TL, Koskimäki J. Incidence of nocturia in 50 to 80-year-old Finnish men. J Urol. 2006;176(6 Pt 1):2541–5. discussion 2545.
48. Viktrup L. The risk of lower urinary tract symptoms five years after the first delivery. Neurourol Urodyn. 2002;21(1):2–29.
49. Viktrup L, Lose G. Incidence and remission of lower urinary tract symptoms during 12 years after the first delivery: a cohort study. J Urol. 2008;180(3):992–7.
50. Häkkinen JT, Shiri R, Koskimäki J, Tammela TL, Auvinen A, Hakama M. Depressive symptoms increase the incidence of nocturia: Tampere Aging Male Urologic Study (TAMUS). J Urol. 2008;179(5):1897–901.
51. Shiri R, Hakama M, Häkkinen J, et al. The effects of lifestyle factors on the incidence of nocturia. J Urol. 2008;180(5):2059–62.
52. Asplund R, Aberg HE. Nocturia in relation to body mass index, smoking and some other life-style factors in women. Climacteric. 2004;7(3):267–73.
53. Fitzgerald MP, Litman HJ, Link CL, McKinlay JB. BACH Survey Investigators. The association of nocturia with cardiac disease, diabetes, body mass index, age and diuretic use: results from the BACH survey. J Urol. 2007;177(4):1385–9.
54. DuBeau CE, Yalla SV, Resnick NM. Implications of the most bothersome prostatism symptom for clinical care and outcomes research. J Am Geriatr Soc. 1995;43(9):985–92.
55. Eckhardt MD, van Venrooij GE, van Melick HH, Boon TA. Prevalence and bothersomeness of lower urinary tract symptoms in benign prostatic hyperplasia and their impact on well-being. J Urol. 2001;166(2):563–8.
56. Swithinbank LV, Donovan JL, du Heaume JC, et al. Urinary symptoms and incontinence in women: relationships between occurrence, age, and perceived impact. Br J Gen Pract. 1999;49(448):897–900.
57. Asplund R, Aberg H. Health of the elderly with regard to sleep and nocturnal micturition. Scand J Prim Health Care. 1992;10(2):98–104.
58. Asplund R, Aberg H. Nocturnal micturition, sleep and well-being in women of ages 40–64 years. Maturitas. 1996;24(1–2):73–81.

59. Ushijima S, Ukimura O, Okihara K, Mizutani Y, Kawauchi A, Miki T. Visual analog scale questionnaire to assess quality of life specific to each symptom of the International Prostate Symptom Score. J Urol. 2006;176(2):665–71.
60. Paunio T, Korhonen T, Hublin C, et al. Longitudinal study on poor sleep and life dissatisfaction in a nationwide cohort of twins. Am J Epidemiol. 2009;169(2):206–13.
61. King CR, Knutson KL, Rathouz PJ, Sidney S, Liu K, Lauderdale DS. Short sleep duration and incident coronary artery calcification. JAMA. 2008;300(24):2859–66.
62. Hublin C, Partinen M, Koskenvuo M, Kaprio J. Sleep and mortality: a population-based 22-year follow-up study. Sleep. 2007;30(10):1245–53.
63. Hetta J. The impact of sleep deprivation caused by nocturia. BJU Int. 1999;84 Suppl 1:27–8.
64. Wagg A, Andersson KE, Cardozo L, et al. Nocturia: morbidity and management in adults. Int J Clin Pract. 2005;59(8):938–45.
65. Middelkoop HA, Smilde-van den Doel DA, Neven AK, Kamphuisen HA, Springer CP. Subjective sleep characteristics of 1,485 males and females aged 50–93: effects of sex and age, and factors related to self-evaluated quality of sleep. J Gerontol A Biol Sci Med Sci. 1996;51(3):M108–15.
66. Bing MH, Moller LA, Jennum P, Mortensen S, Skovgaard LT, Lose G. Prevalence and bother of nocturia, and causes of sleep interruption in a Danish population of men and women aged 60–80 years. BJU Int. 2006;98(3):599–604.
67. Bliwise DL, Foley DJ, Vitiello MV, Ansari FP, Ancoli-Israel S, Walsh JK. Nocturia and disturbed sleep in the elderly. Sleep Med. 2009;10(5):540–8.
68. Pressman MR, Figueroa WG, Kendrick-Mohamed J, Greenspon LW, Peterson DD. Nocturia. A rarely recognized symptom of sleep apnea and other occult sleep disorders. Arch Intern Med. 1996;156(5):545–50.
69. Sagnier PP, MacFarlane G, Teillac P, Botto H, Richard F, Boyle P. Impact of symptoms of prostatism on level of bother and quality of life of men in the French community. J Urol. 1995;153(3 Pt 1):669–73.
70. Liew LC, Tiong HY, Wong ML, Png DC, Tan JK. A population study of nocturia in Singapore. BJU Int. 2006;97(1):109–12.
71. Lowenstein L, Brubaker L, Kenton K, Kramer H, Shott S, FitzGerald MP. Prevalence and impact of nocturia in a urogynecologic population. Int Urogynecol J Pelvic Floor Dysfunct. 2007;18(9):1049–52.
72. Chen FY, Dai YT, Liu CK, Yu HJ, Liu CY, Chen TH. Perception of nocturia and medical consulting behavior among community-dwelling women. Int Urogynecol J Pelvic Floor Dysfunct. 2007;18(4):431–6.
73. Asplund R, Henriksson S, Johansson S, Isacsson G. Nocturia and depression. BJU Int. 2004;93(9):1253–6.
74. Sintonen H. The 15D instrument of health-related quality of life: properties and applications. Ann Med. 2001;33(5):328–36.
75. Olde Rikkert MG, Rigaud AS, van Hoeyweghen RJ, de Graaf J. Geriatric syndromes: medical misnomer or progress in geriatrics? Neth J Med. 2003;61(3):83–7.
76. Järvinen TL, Sievänen H, Khan KM, Heinonen A, Kannus P. Shifting the focus in fracture prevention from osteoporosis to falls. BMJ. 2008;336(7636):124–6.
77. Stewart RB, Moore MT, May FE, Marks RG, Hale WE. Nocturia: a risk factor for falls in the elderly. J Am Geriatr Soc. 1992;40(12):1217–20.
78. Brown JS, Vittinghoff E, Wyman JF, et al. Urinary incontinence: does it increase risk for falls and fractures? Study of Osteoporotic Fractures Research Group. J Am Geriatr Soc. 2000;48(7):721–5.
79. Temml C, Ponholzer A, Gutjahr G, Berger I, Marszalek M, Madersbacher S. Nocturia is an age-independent risk factor for hip-fractures in men. Neurourol Urodyn. 2009;28(8):949–52.
80. Asplund R. Hip fractures, nocturia, and nocturnal polyuria in the elderly. Arch Gerontol Geriatr. 2006;43(3):319–26.

81. Parsons JK, Mougey J, Lambert L, et al. Lower urinary tract symptoms increase the risk of falls in older men. BJU Int. 2009;104(1):63–8.
82. Vaughan CP, Brown CJ, Goode PS, Burgio KL, Allman RM, Johnson 2nd TM. The association of nocturia with incident falls in an elderly community-dwelling cohort. Int J Clin Pract. 2010;64(5):577–83.
83. Nakagawa H, Niu K, Hozawa A, et al. Impact of nocturia on bone fracture and mortality in older individuals: a Japanese longitudinal cohort study. J Urol. 2010;184(4):1413–8.
84. Asplund R. Mortality in the elderly in relation to nocturnal micturition. BJU Int. 1999;84(3):297–301.
85. Bursztyn M, Jacob J, Stessman J. Usefulness of nocturia as a mortality risk factor for coronary heart disease among persons born in 1920 or 1921. Am J Cardiol. 2006;98(10):1311–5.
86. Guyatt GH, Sackett DL, Sinclair JC, Hayward R, Cook DJ, Cook RJ. Users' guides to the medical literature. IX. A method for grading health care recommendations. Evidence-Based Medicine Working Group. JAMA. 1995;274(22):1800–4.
87. Schunemann HJ, Oxman AD, Brozek J, et al. Grading quality of evidence and strength of recommendations for diagnostic tests and strategies. BMJ. 2008;336(7653):1106–10.
88. Tikkinen KA, Auvinen A, Johnson 2nd TM, et al. A systematic evaluation of factors associated with nocturia – the population-based FINNO study. Am J Epidemiol. 2009;170(3):361–8.
89. Yu HJ, Chen TH, Chie WC, Liu CY, Tung TH, Huang SW. Prevalence and associated factors of nocturia among adult residents of the Matsu area of Taiwan. J Formos Med Assoc. 2005;104(6):444–7.
90. Homma Y, Yamaguchi T, Kondo Y, Horie S, Takahashi S, Kitamura T. Significance of nocturia in the International Prostate Symptom Score for benign prostatic hyperplasia. J Urol. 2002;167(1):172–6.
91. Yoshimura K, Ohara H, Ichioka K, et al. Nocturia and benign prostatic hyperplasia. Urology. 2003;61(4):786–90.
92. Johnson 2nd TM, Burrows PK, Kusek JW, et al. The effect of doxazosin, finasteride and combination therapy on nocturia in men with benign prostatic hyperplasia. J Urol. 2007;178(5):2045–50, discussion 2050–1.
93. Abrams PH, Farrar DJ, Turner-Warwick RT, Whiteside CG, Feneley RC. The results of prostatectomy: a symptomatic and urodynamic analysis of 152 patients. J Urol. 1979;121(5):640–2.
94. Bruskewitz RC, Larsen EH, Madsen PO, Dorflinger T. 3-year followup of urinary symptoms after transurethral resection of the prostate. J Urol. 1986;136(3):613–5.
95. Bech P, Rasmussen NA, Olsen LR, Noerholm V, Abildgaard W. The sensitivity and specificity of the Major Depression Inventory, using the Present State Examination as the index of diagnostic validity. J Affect Disord. 2001;66(2–3):159–64.
96. Asplund R, Johansson S, Henriksson S, Isacsson G. Nocturia, depression and antidepressant medication. BJU Int. 2005;95(6):820–3.
97. McKeigue PM, Reynard JM. Relation of nocturnal polyuria of the elderly to essential hypertension. Lancet. 2000;355(9202):486–8.
98. Bulpitt CJ, Connor M, Schulte M, Fletcher AE. Bisoprolol and nifedipine retard in elderly hypertensive patients: effect on quality of life. J Hum Hypertens. 2000;14(3):205–12.
99. Reynard JM, Cannon A, Yang Q, Abrams P. A novel therapy for nocturnal polyuria: a double-blind randomized trial of frusemide against placebo. Br J Urol. 1998;81(2):215–8.
100. Gourova LW, van de Beek C, Spigt MG, Nieman FH, van Kerrebroeck PE. Predictive factors for nocturia in elderly men: a cross-sectional study in 21 general practices. BJU Int. 2006;97(3):528–32.
101. Compston A, Coles A. Multiple sclerosis. Lancet. 2002;359(9313):1221–31.
102. Ouslander JG. Management of overactive bladder. N Engl J Med. 2004;350(8):786–99.
103. Winge K, Fowler CJ. Bladder dysfunction in Parkinsonism: mechanisms, prevalence, symptoms, and management. Mov Disord. 2006;21(6):737–45.

104. DasGupta R, Fowler CJ. Bladder, bowel and sexual dysfunction in multiple sclerosis: management strategies. Drugs. 2003;63(2):153–66.
105. Asplund R. Nocturia in relation to sleep, somatic diseases and medical treatment in the elderly. BJU Int. 2002;90(6):533–6.
106. Partinen M. Sleep disorder related to Parkinson's disease. J Neurol. 1997;244(4 Suppl 1):S3–6.
107. Young A, Home M, Churchward T, Freezer N, Holmes P, Ho M. Comparison of sleep disturbance in mild versus severe Parkinson's disease. Sleep. 2002;25(5):573–7.
108. Hornyak M, Kopasz M, Berger M, Riemann D, Voderholzer U. Impact of sleep-related complaints on depressive symptoms in patients with restless legs syndrome. J Clin Psychiatry. 2005;66(9):1139–45.
109. Pearson VE, Gamaldo CE, Allen RP, Lesage S, Hening WA, Earley CJ. Medication use in patients with restless legs syndrome compared with a control population. Eur J Neurol. 2008;15(1):16–21.
110. Abrams P, Cardozo L, Fall M, et al. The standardisation of terminology of lower urinary tract function: report from the Standardisation Sub-committee of the International Continence Society. Neurourol Urodyn. 2002;21(2):167–78.
111. Blanker MH, Bernsen RM, Ruud Bosch JL, et al. Normal values and determinants of circadian urine production in older men: a population based study. J Urol. 2002;168(4 Pt 1):1453–7.
112. Torimoto K, Hirayama A, Samma S, Yoshida K, Fujimoto K, Hirao Y. The relationship between nocturnal polyuria and the distribution of body fluid: assessment by bioelectric impedance analysis. J Urol. 2009;181(1):219–24. discussion 224.
113. Sugaya K, Nishijima S, Owan T, Oda M, Miyazato M, Ogawa Y. Effects of walking exercise on nocturia in the elderly. Biomed Res. 2007;28(2):101–5.
114. Asplund R. The nocturnal polyuria syndrome (NPS). Gen Pharmacol. 1995;26(6):1203–9.
115. Miller M. Nocturnal polyuria in older people: pathophysiology and clinical implications. J Am Geriatr Soc. 2000;48(10):1321–9.
116. Weiss JP, Blaivas JG. Nocturnal polyuria versus overactive bladder in nocturia. Urology. 2002;60(5 Suppl 1):28–32. discussion 32.
117. Laven BA, Orsini N, Andersson SO, Johansson JE, Gerber GS, Wolk A. Birth weight, abdominal obesity and the risk of lower urinary tract symptoms in a population based study of Swedish men. J Urol. 2008;179(5):1891–5. discussion 1895–6.
118. Bing MH, Moller LA, Jennum P, Mortensen S, Lose G. Nocturia and associated morbidity in a Danish population of men and women aged 60–80 years. BJU Int. 2008;102(7):808–14.
119. Subak LL, Wing R, West DS, et al. Weight loss to treat urinary incontinence in overweight and obese women. N Engl J Med. 2009;360(5):481–90.
120. Lee WC, Wu HP, Tai TY, Liu SP, Chen J, Yu HJ. Effects of diabetes on female voiding behavior. J Urol. 2004;172(3):989–92.
121. Fitzgerald MP, Mulligan M, Parthasarathy S. Nocturic frequency is related to severity of obstructive sleep apnea, improves with continuous positive airways treatment. Am J Obstet Gynecol. 2006;194(5):1399–403.
122. Sarma AV, Burke JP, Jacobson DJ, et al. Associations between diabetes and clinical markers of benign prostatic hyperplasia among community-dwelling Black and White men. Diabetes Care. 2008;31(3):476–82.
123. Abrams P, Artibani W, Cardozo L, et al. Reviewing the ICS 2002 terminology report: the ongoing debate. Neurourol Urodyn. 2009;28(4):287.
124. Wein AJ, Rackley RR. Overactive bladder: a better understanding of pathophysiology, diagnosis and management. J Urol. 2006;175(3 Pt 2):S5–10.
125. Krystal AD, Preud'homme XA, Amundsen CL, Webster GD. Detrusor overactivity persisting at night and preceding nocturia in patients with overactive bladder syndrome: a nocturnal cystometrogram and polysomnogram study. J Urol. 2010;184(2):623–8.
126. Matharu G, Donaldson MM, McGrother CW, Matthews RJ. Relationship between urinary symptoms reported in a postal questionnaire and urodynamic diagnosis. Neurourol Urodyn. 2005;24(2):100–5.

127. Tikkinen KA, Tammela TL, Rissanen AM, Valpas A, Huhtala H, Auvinen A. Is the prevalence of overactive bladder overestimated? A population-based study in Finland. PLoS One. 2007;2:e195.
128. Michel MC, de la Rosette JJ. Role of muscarinic receptor antagonists in urgency and nocturia. BJU Int. 2005;96 Suppl 1:37–42.
129. Brown CT, O'Flynn E, Van Der Meulen J, Newman S, Mundy AR, Emberton M. The fear of prostate cancer in men with lower urinary tract symptoms: should symptomatic men be screened? BJU Int. 2003;91(1):30–2.
130. Chapter 1: Diagnosis and Treatment Recommendations. In: Guideline on the Management of Benign Prostatic Hyperplasia (BPH). American Urological Association Education and Research, Inc. http://www.auanet.org/content/guidelines-and-quality-care/clinical-guidelines/main-reports/bph-management/chapt_1_appendix.pdf (2003). Accessed 2 Feb 2011.
131. Young JM, Muscatello DJ, Ward JE. Are men with lower urinary tract symptoms at increased risk of prostate cancer? A systematic review and critique of the available evidence. BJU Int. 2000;85(9):1037–48.
132. Damber JE, Aus G. Prostate cancer. Lancet. 2008;371(9625):1710–21.
133. Sanda MG, Dunn RL, Michalski J, et al. Quality of life and satisfaction with outcome among prostate-cancer survivors. N Engl J Med. 2008;358(12):1250–61.
134. Namiki S, Saito S, Ishidoya S, et al. Adverse effect of radical prostatectomy on nocturia and voiding frequency symptoms. Urology. 2005;66(1):147–51.
135. Namiki S, Ishidoya S, Saito S, et al. Natural history of voiding function after radical retropubic prostatectomy. Urology. 2006;68(1):142–7.
136. Martin RM, Vatten L, Gunnell D, Romundstad P, Nilsen TI. Lower urinary tract symptoms and risk of prostate cancer: the HUNT 2 Cohort, Norway. Int J Cancer. 2008;123(8):1924–8.
137. Klein BE, Klein R, Lee KE, Bruskewitz RC. Correlates of urinary symptom scores in men. Am J Public Health. 1999;89(11):1745–8.
138. Hsieh CH, Chen HY, Hsu CS, Chang ST, Chiang CD. Risk factors for nocturia in Taiwanese women aged 20–59 years. Taiwan J Obstet Gynecol. 2007;46(2):166–70.
139. Kang D, Andriole GL, Van De Vooren RC, et al. Risk behaviours and benign prostatic hyperplasia. BJU Int. 2004;93(9):1241–5.
140. Shaper AG, Wannamethee G, Walker M. Alcohol and mortality in British men: explaining the U-shaped curve. Lancet. 1988;2(8623):1267–73.
141. Fillmore KM, Stockwell T, Chikritzhs T, Bostrom A, Kerr W. Moderate alcohol use and reduced mortality risk: systematic error in prospective studies and new hypotheses. Ann Epidemiol. 2007;17(5 Suppl):S16–23.
142. Naimi TS, Brown DW, Brewer RD, et al. Cardiovascular risk factors and confounders among nondrinking and moderate-drinking U.S. adults. Am J Prev Med. 2005;28(4):369–73.
143. Jackson R, Broad J, Connor J, Wells S. Alcohol and ischaemic heart disease: probably no free lunch. Lancet. 2005;366(9501):1911–2.
144. Platz EA, Kawachi I, Rimm EB, et al. Physical activity and benign prostatic hyperplasia. Arch Intern Med. 1998;158(21):2349–56.
145. Prezioso D, Catuogno C, Galassi P, D'Andrea G, Castello G, Pirritano D. Life-style in patients with LUTS suggestive of BPH. Eur Urol. 2001;40 Suppl 1:9–12.
146. Rohrmann S, Crespo CJ, Weber JR, Smit E, Giovannucci E, Platz EA. Association of cigarette smoking, alcohol consumption and physical activity with lower urinary tract symptoms in older American men: findings from the third National Health and Nutrition Examination Survey. BJU Int. 2005;96(1):77–82.
147. Soda T, Masui K, Okuno H, Terai A, Ogawa O, Yoshimura K. Efficacy of nondrug lifestyle measures for the treatment of nocturia. J Urol. 2010;184(3):1000–4.
148. Kupelian V, Link CL, Hall SA, McKinlay JB. Are racial/ethnic disparities in the prevalence of nocturia due to socioeconomic status? Results of the BACH Survey. J Urol. 2009;181(4):1756.
149. Burgio KL, Johnson 2nd TM, Goode PS, et al. Prevalence and correlates of nocturia in community-dwelling older adults. J Am Geriatr Soc. 2010;58(5):861–6.

150. Markland AD, Vaughan CP, Johnson 2nd TM, Goode PS, Redden DT, Burgio KL. Prevalence of nocturia in United States men: results from the National Health and Nutrition Examination Survey. J Urol. 2011;185(3):998–1002.
151. Gopal M, Sammel MD, Pien G, et al. Investigating the associations between nocturia and sleep disorders in perimenopausal women. J Urol. 2008;180(5):2063–7.
152. Munro-Faure AD, Beilin LJ, Bulpitt CJ, et al. Comparison of black and white patients attending hypertension clinics in England. Br Med J. 1979;1(6170):1044–7.
153. Sze EH, Jones WP, Ferguson JL, Barker CD, Dolezal JM. Prevalence of urinary incontinence symptoms among black, white, and Hispanic women. Obstet Gynecol. 2002;99(4):572–5.
154. Kuo HC. Prevalence of lower urinary tract symptoms in male aborigines and non-aborigines in eastern Taiwan. J Formos Med Assoc. 2008;107(9):728–35.
155. Chuang FC, Kuo HC. Prevalence of lower urinary tract symptoms in indigenous and non-indigenous women in Eastern Taiwan. J Formos Med Assoc. 2010;109(3):228–36.
156. Mariappan P, Turner KJ, Sothilingam S, Rajan P, Sundram M, Stewart LH. Nocturia, nocturia indices and variables from frequency-volume charts are significantly different in Asian and Caucasian men with lower urinary tract symptoms: a prospective comparison study. BJU Int. 2007;100(2):332–6.
157. Lose G, Alling-Moller L, Jennum P. Nocturia in women. Am J Obstet Gynecol. 2001;185(2):514–21.
158. Allsworth JE, Omicioli VA, Cunkelman JA, Homco J. Reproductive factors associated with nocturia and urgency: Tikkinen et al. Am J Obstet Gynecol. 2008;199(2):205–6.
159. Aslan D, Aslan G, Yamazhan M, Ispahi C, Tinar S. Voiding symptoms in pregnancy: an assessment with international prostate symptom score. Gynecol Obstet Invest. 2003;55(1):46–9.
160. Parboosingh J, Doig A. Studies of nocturia in normal pregnancy. J Obstet Gynaecol Br Commonw. 1973;80(10):888–95.
161. Tikkinen KA, Auvinen A, Tiitinen A, Valpas A, Johnson 2nd TM, Tammela TL. Reproductive factors associated with nocturia and urinary urgency in women – a population-based study in Finland. Am J Obstet Gynecol. 2008;199(2):153.e1–12.
162. Alling Moller L, Lose G, Jorgensen T. Risk factors for lower urinary tract symptoms in women 40 to 60 years of age. Obstet Gynecol. 2000;96(3):446–51.
163. Asplund R, Aberg HE. Development of nocturia in relation to health, age and the menopause. Maturitas. 2005;51(4):358–62.
164. Moline ML, Broch L, Zak R, Gross V. Sleep in women across the life cycle from adulthood through menopause. Sleep Med Rev. 2003;7(2):155–77.
165. Rekers H, Drogendijk AC, Valkenburg HA, Riphagen F. The menopause, urinary incontinence and other symptoms of the genito-urinary tract. Maturitas. 1992;15(2):101–11.
166. Lin TL, Ng SC, Chen YC, Hu SW, Chen GD. What affects the occurrence of nocturia more: menopause or age? Maturitas. 2005;50(2):71–7.
167. Cardozo L, Rekers H, Tapp A, et al. Oestriol in the treatment of postmenopausal urgency: a multicentre study. Maturitas. 1993;18(1):47–53.
168. Liapis A, Bakas P, Georgantopoulou C, Creatsas G. The use of oestradiol therapy in postmenopausal women after TVT-O anti-incontinence surgery. Maturitas. 2010;66(1):101–6.
169. Thakar R, Ayers S, Clarkson P, Stanton S, Manyonda I. Outcomes after total versus subtotal abdominal hysterectomy. N Engl J Med. 2002;347(17):1318–25.
170. Vervest HA, Kiewiet de Jonge M, Vervest TM, Barents JW, Haspels AA. Micturition symptoms and urinary incontinence after non-radical hysterectomy. Acta Obstet Gynecol Scand. 1988;67(2):141–6.
171. Virtanen H, Makinen J, Tenho T, Kiilholma P, Pitkanen Y, Hirvonen T. Effects of abdominal hysterectomy on urinary and sexual symptoms. Br J Urol. 1993;72(6):868–72.
172. Altman D, Lopez A, Falconer C, Zetterstrom J. The impact of hysterectomy on lower urinary tract symptoms. Int Urogynecol J Pelvic Floor Dysfunct. 2003;14(6):418–23.
173. Prasad M, Sadhukhan M, Tom B, Al-Taher H. The effect of hysterectomy on urinary symptoms and residual bladder volume. J Obstet Gynaecol. 2002;22(5):544–7.

174. Resnick NM. Noninvasive diagnosis of the patient with complex incontinence. Gerontology. 1990;36 Suppl 2:8–18.
175. Weiss JP. Nocturia: "do the math". J Urol. 2006;175(3 Pt 2):S16–8.
176. Kujubu DA, Aboseif SR. An overview of nocturia and the syndrome of nocturnal polyuria in the elderly. Nat Clin Pract Nephrol. 2008;4(8):426–35.
177. Appell RA, Sand PK. Nocturia: etiology, diagnosis, and treatment. Neurourol Urodyn. 2008;27(1):34–9.
178. Schneider T, de la Rosette JJ, Michel MC. Nocturia: a non-specific but important symptom of urological disease. Int J Urol. 2009;16(3):249–56.

Chapter 6
Nocturia and Overactive Bladder

Jerry G. Blaivas and Johnson F. Tsui

Keywords Nocturia • Overactive bladder (OAB) • Urgency • Urgency perception Score • Latchkey syndrome • Micturition • Detrusor overactivity

Introduction

In this chapter, the current knowledge about the relationship between nocturia and OAB is reviewed and directions for future research are discussed. Certain caveats though, should be noted. First, the relation between nocturia and overactive bladder is not well understood and the peer-reviewed literature is sparse; hence, much of what appears is based on the author's observations and research. There are a number of reasons for the paucity of information and this relates to the definition of both conditions. Second, with respect to nocturia, there are no validated instruments that determine: (1) why the patient was awakened, i.e., whether or not he was awakened by an urge to void, (2) why he/she voided (out of convenience, habit, urge, or urgency), and (3) whether they fell back asleep. Third, the definitions for OAB and urgency (the sine qua non for the diagnosis of OAB) are the subject of controversy. Finally, as discussed finely by Tikkinen, there are a number of methodological flaws in epidemiologic research whose details are beyond the scope of this discussion, but should be taken into account because their impact decreases the prevalence of OAB by nearly 50% and influences the prevalence of nocturia [1]. These methodological

J.G. Blaivas, MD (✉)
Department of Urology, Weill Medical College of Cornell University, New York, NY, USA

SUNY Downstate College of Medicine, Brooklyn, NY, USA
e-mail: jblvs@aol.com

J.F. Tsui, BS
SUNY Downstate College of Medicine, Brooklyn, NY, USA

flaws include the duration of time over which the prevalence of the OAB was assessed, the exact inclusion and exclusion criteria, the severity and bother, and systemic flaws such as "herding," "winner's curse," and publication bias. For example, using very strict criteria for OAB, Tikkinen found a prevalence of only about 8% compared to the oft quoted 16–17% that has become the standard figure quoted by most authorities [2, 3].

Ultimately though, in order to evaluate the relationship between nocturia and OAB, better methods are needed to determine whether the patient is awakened by OAB symptoms or by something else and whether the nocturic void was due to OAB or out of convenience before going back to sleep.

Definition of Overactive Bladder

The Standardization Committee of the International Continence Society defines OAB as follows [4]:

> (Urinary) Urgency, with or without urge incontinence, usually with frequency and nocturia, can be described as the overactive bladder syndrome…if there is no proven infection or other obvious pathology.

They further go on to describe urgency as "… the complaint of a sudden compelling desire to pass urine, which is difficult to defer." However, these definitions may be too restrictive, especially insofar as determining the relation between OAB and nocturia. In a study designed to define the sensation of urgency, patients were asked to describe, in their own words, what they meant by urgency [5]. The most common answer was, "If I wait too long, I have trouble getting to the bathroom in time." In fact, only a minority of patients described urgency as a "sudden" event. Based on these data, two distinct types of urgency emerged that may have relevance for determining why a patient voids when awakened from sleep. Type 1 urge was described as an intensification of the normal urge to void and occurred in 69% of patients with OAB. Type 2 urge (31%) was a sudden precipitous urge of a different sensation from the normal urge that more closely conformed to the ICS definition. In patients with type 1 urge, the intensity of the urge to void increases over time and culminates in micturition, whereas, in Type 2 urge, the patient has little or no warning and must rush to the bathroom. The idea that the urge to void can be graded runs counter to ICS doctrine [6], but nevertheless has strong scientific support [7–9]. At least four instruments have been devised and validated that can be used as an anamnestic response or in a contemporaneous diary to determine the extent to which urgency is responsible for micturition [10]. One such instrument, the Urgency Perception Score [7], is depicted in Table 6.1.

Although no specific studies have been done to correlate the UPS grade with the symptoms of urgency, expert opinion suggests that UPS voids of grade 3–4 correspond to OAB or urgency voids [11]. If one accepts these definitions (not all do), then a patient who is awakened by a UPS grade 3 or 4 sensation and then voids, would

Table 6.1 Urgency perception score

What is the reason you usually urinate?
Grade 0: Out of convenience? (No urge)
Grade 1: Mild urge (can hold >1 h)
Grade 2: Moderate urge (can hold >10–60 min)
Grade 3: Severe urge (can hold <10 min)
Grade 4: Desperate urge (must go immediately)

be considered to have nocturia caused by OAB. But what about a patient who is awakened by something other than an urge to void or is awakened and has a UPS grade 1 or 2 void? Is that nocturia due to OAB?

Another confounding factor in the analysis of the relationship between OAB and nocturia is the fact that the ICS definition considers OAB to be a syndrome, with symptoms suggestive of detrusor overactivity (involuntary contractions of the bladder), and recommends that the term OAB be used only "if there is no proven infection or other obvious pathology." This definition has profound effects on research methodology because, in fact, there are a large number of conditions in the differential diagnosis of OAB symptoms that should, theoretically, be exclusion criteria. In practice, however, most studies do not include such exclusion criteria. For example, in two recent studies of the differential diagnosis, OAB was found to be idiopathic in only 5% of men and 23% of women. In men, the following differential diagnosis was reported: benign prostatic enlargement (32%), urethral obstruction (prostatic and stricture) (22%), complications of prostate cancer treatment (20%), neurogenic bladder (11%), idiopathic (5%), bladder stone (2%), and bladder cancer (1%) [12]. In women, 23% had idiopathic OAB. The differential diagnosis in women included stress incontinence (33%), pelvic organ prolapse (24%), bladder outlet obstruction (10%), neurogenic bladder (7%), prior pelvic surgery (6%), bladder cancer (1%) and urethral diverticulum (1%) [13]. In fact, every one of these conditions was proposed by Tikkinen to be risk factors for developing nocturia.

Definition of Nocturia

The definition of nocturia is discussed in great detail in Chap. 1, and also presents conundrums of its own. Central to the problem in defining nocturia is the difference between nocturia and nighttime voiding. Homma suggested that the term nocturia be restricted to voids that occur during sleep time only when they are accompanied by an urge to void [14]. All other voids that occur between going to bed with the intention to go to sleep and rising in the morning are considered nighttime voids (see Fig. 6.1). Although this makes good sense from a scientific standpoint, in clinical practice, the distinction is usually not made. In our experience, patients usually cannot be sure what awakened them – an urge to void or something else and to our knowledge there are no validated instruments capable of clarifying the issue.

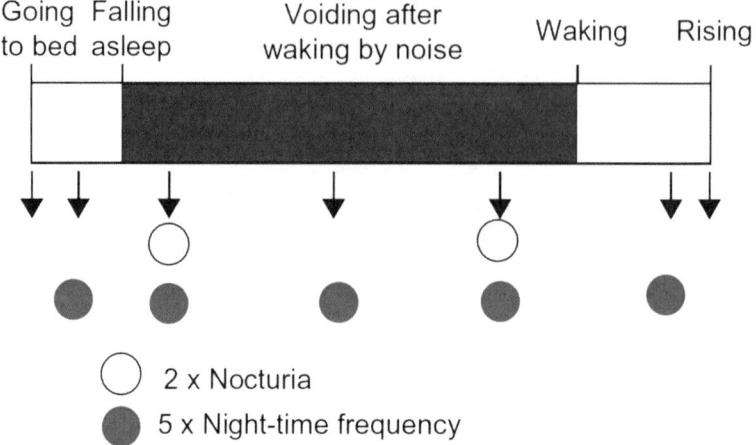

Fig. 6.1 The distinction between nighttime voiding and nocturia. (Figure is reprinted and legend is modified with permission from Homma [14])

Relationship Between OAB and Nocturia

According to the ICS definition, nocturia is one of the cardinal symptoms of OAB and from a clinical standpoint, it is well known that nocturia is common in patients with OAB. Notwithstanding all of the methodological problems engendered by concerns alluded to above, it seems evident from the studies that follow that OAB is a major risk factor in both men and women for having nocturia, but the converse is not true as only about one-third of nocturics have OAB. Tikkinen conducted a Finnish population-based study of 6,000 postal questionnaires that had a 62% response rate (1,670 men and 1,837 women). In this study, the Danish Prostatic Symptom Score (DAN-PSS) and American Urological Association Symptom Score (AUASS) were used to determine the presence of nocturia and a paraphrase of the definition of urgency was used as the proxy for OAB. He reported that one-third of patients with nocturia at least twice a night reported OAB, and, conversely, 40% of women and 56% of men with OAB reported nocturia (defined as at least two voids per night). Furthermore, there was a direct relationship between the number of nocturnal voids and the prevalence of OAB ($p<0.001$). Nocturia and OAB increased with age ($p<0.001$) and this relationship persisted across age groups [1].

Several other studies have shown comparable results with a reported incidence of OAB as high as 33% in patients with nocturia and a 50% incidence of nocturia in those with OAB [15–18].

In an observational study of women with OAB who underwent urodynamics, Matharu reported that in women over 40 years of age, the incidence of detrusor overactivity increased with increasing self-reported nocturia; i.e., the greater the number of nighttime voids, the greater the chance of having DO [19]. The odds ratio ranged from 1.9 for one nighttime void to 3.1 for three nighttime voids.

Indirect evidence that OAB plays a relatively minor role in the genesis of nocturnal voids comes from studies that demonstrate the lack of effectiveness of OAB medications in reducing nighttime voids [20, 21]. However, these studies do suggest that antimuscarinics reduce the number of nighttime voids that occur due to urgency. For example, in a non-placebo-controlled study, Brubaker et al. reported that solifenacin reduced the number of nocturnal voids by 36% in patients without nocturnal polyuria, while having no effect on overall nocturnal voids in patients with nocturnal polyuria [21].

From the studies cited above, we can conclude that: (1) most patients with nocturia do not have OAB, (2) about half of patients with OAB have nocturia, (3) antimuscarinics do not appear to be efficacious for nocturia, and (4) antimuscarinics may be effective for nocturnal voids due to urgency.

Future Directions for Research

The first problem that needs to be addressed is improving the definitions of nocturia and OAB. The problems with both definitions have been discussed in detail above, but until the issues are resolved, it will be difficult to go forward with meaningful research. Once the definitions are worked out, the two most critical problems are determining why the patient awakened in the first place – because of a need to void or something else and whether the need to void was a compelling one (an OAB void) or a convenience void (I'd better void before I go back to sleep so I don't get up later). To compound this further is the possibility of a Pavlovian response once the patient decides to void, gets out of bed and, on the way to the bathroom, develops urgency ("latchkey syndrome") [22].

References

1. Tikkinen KAO. Epidemiology of nocturia: results from the FINNO study. In: Medical School. Tampere: University of Tampere; 2010. p. 222.
2. Milsom I et al. How widespread are the symptoms of an overactive bladder and how are they managed? A population-based prevalence study. BJU Int. 2001;87(9):760–6.
3. Stewart WF et al. Prevalence and burden of overactive bladder in the United States. World J Urol. 2003;20(6):327–36.
4. Abrams P et al. The standardisation of terminology of lower urinary tract function: report from the Standardisation Sub-committee of the International Continence Society. Neurourol Urodyn. 2002;21(2):167–78.
5. Blaivas JG et al. Two types of urgency. Neurourol Urodyn. 2009;28(3):188–90.
6. Chapple CR et al. The role of urinary urgency and its measurement in the overactive bladder symptom syndrome: current concepts and future prospects. BJU Int. 2005;95(3):335–40.
7. Blaivas JG et al. The urgency perception score: validation and test-retest. J Urol. 2007;177(1):199–202.
8. Nixon A et al. A validated patient reported measure of urinary urgency severity in overactive bladder for use in clinical trials. J Urol. 2005;174(2):604–7.

9. Zinner N et al. The overactive bladder-symptom composite score: a composite symptom score of toilet voids, urgency severity and urge urinary incontinence in patients with overactive bladder. J Urol. 2005;173(5):1639–43.
10. Coyne KS et al. Development and validation of patient-reported outcomes measures for overactive bladder: a review of concepts. Urology. 2006;68(2 Suppl):9–16.
11. Guan Z, Harel M, Blaivas JG, Wang J, Weiss JP. Linear Correlation and Regression Between Severity of Urge Sensation and Voided Volume in Subjects With Overactive Bladder: A Different Approach to Understanding Urgency. J Urol. 2010;183(4):Suppl. p. e591.
12. Blaivas JG et al. Differential diagnosis of overactive bladder in men. J Urol. 2009;182(6):2814–7.
13. Marks BK. Differential diagnosis of overactive bladder in women. Valentine Essay Competition, New York Academy of Medicine, April 2011.
14. Homma Y. Lower urinary tract symptomatology: its definition and confusion. Int J Urol. 2008;15(1):35–43.
15. Schatzl G et al. Cross-sectional study of nocturia in both sexes: analysis of a voluntary health screening project. Urology. 2000;56(1):71–5.
16. Rembratt A, Norgaard JP, Andersson KE. Nocturia and associated morbidity in a community-dwelling elderly population. BJU Int. 2003;92(7):726–30.
17. Weiss JP et al. Age related pathogenesis of nocturia in patients with overactive bladder. J Urol. 2007;178(2):548–51. discussion 551.
18. Yoshimura K et al. Prevalence of and risk factors for nocturia: analysis of a health screening program. Int J Urol. 2004;11(5):282–7.
19. Matharu G et al. Relationship between urinary symptoms reported in a postal questionnaire and urodynamic diagnosis. Neurourol Urodyn. 2005;24(2):100–5.
20. Rackley R et al. Nighttime dosing with tolterodine reduces overactive bladder-related nocturnal micturitions in patients with overactive bladder and nocturia. Urology. 2006;67(4):731–6. discussion 736.
21. Brubaker L, FitzGerald MP. Nocturnal polyuria and nocturia relief in patients treated with solifenacin for overactive bladder symptoms. Int Urogynecol J Pelvic Floor Dysfunct. 2007;18(7):737–41.
22. Ghei M, Malone-Lee J. Using the circumstances of symptom experience to assess the severity of urgency in the overactive bladder. J Urol. 2005;174(3):972–6.

Chapter 7
Nocturia and Surgical Treatment of the Prostate

David D. Thiel and Steven P. Petrou

Keywords Lower urinary tract symptoms (LUTS) • Benign Prostatic Hyperplasia (BPH) • Transurethral resection of the prostate (TURP) • American Urologic Association Symptom score (AUASS) • International Consultation on Incontinence Nocturia Quality of Life (NQOL) • Hours of uninterrupted sleep (HUS) • Radical prostatectomy (RP)

Lower urinary tract symptoms (LUTS) suggestive of benign prostatic hyperplasia (BPH) are common in the aging male [1]. The incidence of nocturia increases with age as well, with rates ranging from 30% of men over 50 years of age to 60% of men in their 70s [2]. Nocturia has been noted to be the most bothersome symptom in men with LUTS suspected of or having BPH [3]. Multivariate analysis has shown that nocturia is one of the most important factors determining pretreatment health-related quality of life (HRQOL) in patients with BPH/LUTS [4].

Bladder outlet procedures such as transurethral resection of the prostate (TURP), used to treat LUTS associated with BPH, will improve obstructive symptoms. The effect of outlet procedures on storage symptoms such as nocturia has been more difficult to delineate. Confounding analysis is that as patients age, nocturia may have multiple etiologies, both urologic and nonurologic [5]. Therefore, nocturia will persist in a significant proportion of patients following outlet procedures. The lack of randomized trials comparing outcomes of bladder outlet procedures to medical therapy as well as technique-based studies (TURP vs. laser vs. microwave therapy, etc.) combined with the lack metrics that assess nocturia as an individual outcome of invasive outlet procedures make it difficult to delineate the true impact of prostate surgery on nocturia.

D.D. Thiel, MD • S.P. Petrou, MD (✉)
Department of Urology, Mayo Clinic, Jacksonville, FL, USA
e-mail: petrou.steven@mayo.edu

Metrics for Evaluation of Outcomes of Outlet Procedures in Men with BPH and Nocturia

The proper assessment and epidemiology of nocturia in patients with LUTS were traditionally difficult to define because most questionnaires included nocturia in one or more items, among the other LUTS [3]. Nocturia is included as one of several items which are added together to form a score (e.g., IPSS [6], BPH impact index [7], etc.). Very few instruments examine the impact of nocturia alone on quality of life. Quality of life is linked with the WHO definition of health which refers to a state of physical, emotional, and social well-being and not just the absence of disease [8]. Nocturia itself affects overall QOL by affecting general health and, sleep continuity, causing a condition of worry about the need to wake to urinate, and may even have relation to mortality [9].

IPSS/AUASS

The American Urologic Association Symptom score (AUASS) (Table 7.1) is a validated self-report questionnaire that assesses the severity of LUTS associated with the prostate [10]. It contains seven items, each with a response scale with six choices ranging from 0 (no symptoms) to 5 (symptoms always present) [10]. Summation of the scores allows for classification of LUTS as mild (total score, 0 to 7), moderate (total score, 8–19), and severe (total score 20–35). The International Prostate Symptom Score (IPSS) is the same as the AUASS with an additional question designed to assess the degree of "bother" associated with the patient's urinary symptoms (0, delighted to 6, terrible).

The symptoms that are graded are not specific to the prostate and can also be seen in women. Scores do not correlate with urodynamic indices such as the degree of bladder outlet obstruction or detrusor overactivity [11–13]. The IPSS also does not delineate the effect of nocturia upon sleep quality or how decreasing sleep quality affects quality of life [6]. The IPSS does not capture the full morbidity of the voiding problem experienced by the individual patient in their daily life. However, it acts as a good screening tool to assess symptom bother and serves as a pre-intervention measurement (prior to medical therapy or surgery) to assess therapeutic outcomes.

BPH Impact Index [7]

The BPH impact index (Table 7.2) was an attempt by Barry et al. in 1995 to develop a more concise questionnaire to evaluate the degree to which LUTS impacted patient's quality of life or was bothersome for them. It is a self-administered

7 Nocturia and Surgical Treatment of the Prostate

Table 7.1 American Urologic Association Symptom Score (or the International Prostate Symptom Score) [10]

AUA symptom index for BPH

	Not at all	Less than 1 time in 5	Less than half the time	About half the time	More than half the time	Almost always
1. Over the past month, how often have you had a sensation of not emptying your bladder completely after you finish urinating?	0	1	2	3	4	5
2. Over the past month, how often have you had to urinate again less than 2 hours after you finished urinating?	0	1	2	3	4	5
3. Over the past month, how often have you found you stopped and started again several times when you urinated?	0	1	2	3	4	5
4. Over the past month, how often have you found it difficult to postpone urination?	0	1	2	3	4	5
5. Over the past month, how often have you had a weak urinary stream?	0	1	2	3	4	5
6. Over the past month, how often have you had to push or strain to begin urination?	0	1	2	3	4	5
7. Over the last month, how many times did you most typically get up to urinate form the time you went to bed at night until you got up in the morning?	None 0	1 time 1	2 times 2	3 times 3	4 times 4	5 or more times 5

Score = sum of questions 1–7 =

Table 7.2 Benign prostatic hyperplasia impact index [7]

BPH impact index

1. Over the past month, how much physical discomfort did any urinary problems cause you?
  0 ___ None
  1 ___ Only a little
  2 ___ Some
  3 ___ A lot

2. Over the past month, how much did you worry about your health because of any urinary problems?
  0 ___ None
  1 ___ Only a little
  2 ___ Some
  3 ___ A lot

3. Overall, how bothersome has any trouble with urination been during the past month?
  0 ___ Not at all bothersome
  1 ___ Bothers me a little
  2 ___ Bothers me some
  3 ___ Bothers me a lot

4. Over the past month, how much of the time has any urinary problems kept you from doing the kinds of things you would usually do?
  0 ___ Not at all bothersome
  1 ___ Bothers me a little
  2 ___ Bothers me some
  3 ___ Bothers me a lot

BPH Impact Score = sum of questions 1–4 = _____

four-item questionnaire with scores ranging from 0 to 12 (higher scores indicating more severe symptoms and poorer quality of life). The questions measure aspects of physical discomfort, worry, bother, and interference with everyday activities.

Barry et al. defined five global ratings of symptom improvement with regard to IPSS and BPH impact index [14]. The five ratings are "markedly improved," "moderately improved," "slightly improved," "unchanged," or "worse." The goal of this instrument is to determine how much of a change in symptom scores is perceptible to patients. This rating system is designed to provide the data required to determine sample sizes and clinical significance of symptom improvement in BPH clinical trials [15].

NQOL

The International Consultation on Incontinence Nocturia Quality of Life (NQOL) was first described by Abraham in 2004 and was the initial validated instrument that examined the QOL impact of nocturia alone [16]. The NQOL is a 13-item questionnaire with 12 items related directly to nocturia and one to general QOL (Table 7.3). The questions cover factors of daytime energy, worry, productivity, sleep, and vitality. The 12 items pertaining to nocturia are scored from 0 (no symptoms) to

Table 7.3 Nocturia quality of life questionaire [16]

Over the past 2 weeks, having to get up at night to urinate…					
1. Has made it difficult for me to concentrate the next day	☐ Every day	☐ Most days	☐ Some days	☐ Rarely	☐ Never
2. Has made me feel generally low in energy the next day	☐ Every day	☐ Most days	☐ Some days	☐ Rarely	☐ Never
3. Has required me to nape during the day	☐ Every day	☐ Most days	☐ Some days	☐ Rarely	☐ Never
4. Has made me less productive the next day	☐ Every day	☐ Most days	☐ Some days	☐ Rarely	☐ Never
5. Has caused me to participate less in activities I enjoy	☐ Extremely	☐ Quite a bit	☐ Moderately	☐ A little bit	☐ Not at all
6. Has caused me to be careful about when or how much I drink	☐ All the time	☐ Most of the time	☐ Some of the time	☐ Rarely	☐ Never
7. Has made it difficult for me to get enough sleep at night	☐ Every night	☐ Most nights	☐ Some nights	☐ Rarely	☐ Never
Over the past 2 weeks, i have been……..					
8. Concerned that I am disturbing others in the house because of having to get up at night to urinate	☐ Extremely	☐ Quite a bit	☐ Moderately	☐ A little bit	☐ Not at all
9. Preoccupied about having to get up at night to urinate	☐ All the time	☐ Most of the time	☐ Some of the time	☐ Rarely	☐ Never
10. Worried that this condition will get worse in the future	☐ Extremely	☐ Quite a bit	☐ Moderately	☐ A little bit	☐ Not at all
11. Worried that there is no effective treatment for this condition (having to get up at night to urinate)	☐ Extremely	☐ Quite a bit	☐ Moderately	☐ A little bit	☐ Not at all
12. Overall, how bothersome has having to get up at night to urinate been during the past 2 weeks?	☐ Not at all	☐ A little bit	☐ Moderately	☐ Quite a bit	☐ Extremely
13. Overall I would rate my quality of life to be…	☐ Very Good	☐ Good	☐ Fair	☐ Poor	☐ Very Poor

4 (symptoms always present). The 13th item related to quality of life is scored from 0 (no symptoms) to 10 (severe nocturia impact on QOL) [3, 16]. The questionnaire takes approximately 5 min to fill out and scores range from 0 to 48 [16]. The authors found the NQOL to have good internal consistency (using Cronbach's alpha coefficient [17]), test–retest reliability, and convergent validity with the PSQI and SF-36 (see paragraph below).

Cai et al. [3] validated the NQOL in an Italian population of 111 men (61 affected with BPH/LUTS undergoing outlet surgery and 48 controls). The IPSS was used to validate the effect of LUTS on quality of life and the PSQI (Pittsburgh Sleep Quality Index) was used to measure sleep quality [18]. The ESS (Epworth Sleepiness Scale) was used to measure daytime sleepiness in the surgical patients [19]. The NQOL was found to have good convergent validity with IPSS, PSQI, and ESS. Internal consistency was high and there was good test–retest reliability [3]. The NQOL also had good sensitivity for changes in assessments before and after outlet procedures. Others have stressed the importance of using the NQOL to specifically measure nocturia after discovering that NQOL scores do not correlate with the IPSS prior to outlet procedures and are not associated with NQOL improvement following prostatectomy [20]. Each instrument has its own limitations and critics of the NQOL point out that although the measure has reasonable content validity, it does not contain items related to elderly patients such as feeling older from the fear of falling associated with nocturia [21].

HUS

Hours of uninterrupted sleep (HUS) is a helpful metric to assess the affect of nocturia on the quality of sleep [22]. HUS is defined as the time from falling asleep to the first wakening to void. Deep slow-wave restorative sleep occurs most often during the first hours of the night, while lighter, less restorative sleep dominates the second part of the night [23]. It is thought that waking during deep sleep most likely contributes to daytime fatigue; consequently, quality of sleep is affected not only by nighttime voiding frequency but also by the actual time of waking to void [20]. By way of example, drug trials for tamsulosin have validated that decreases in nighttime voiding frequency correlate with increases in HUS and quality of life [24].

Surgical Therapy of the Prostate and Nocturia

In patients with LUTS suggestive of BPH, nocturia is thought to be caused by a variable combination of elevated postvoid residuals, nocturnal polyuria, detrusor overactivity, and low functional bladder capacity [16, 20]. The contribution of other etiologies of nocturia, besides LUTS/BPH, may alter the apparent efficacy of surgical treatments with regard to specific nocturia improvement. Studies examining the effect of outlet procedures on nocturia typically focus on question #7 of the IPSS: "during the last month, how many times did you most typically get up to urinate from the time you went to bed at night until the time you got up in the morning?" [4] These types of univariate analyses are less valid than those utilizing multiple regression approaches to investigate the outcomes of therapy with regard to nocturia in the presence of multiple explanatory variables [4]. However, large samples of patients are required to maintain statistical power in multivariate analysis.

Radical Prostatectomy and nocturia

Radical prostatectomy (RP) for prostate cancer is associated with improvement in IPSS scores in patients with values in the moderate or severe range. [25]. Lepor et al. noted mean AUA symptom scores decreased by 51% 12 months following RP. There was a statistical improvement following surgery in all questions in the index except for question #7 of the IPSS (nocturia question). A 2005 study evaluating 120 patients following RP also noted improvement in all urinary indices except nocturia in patients with moderate or severe IPSS scores [26]. The patients were divided into three groups based on their preoperative nocturia symptom scores (again, question #7). N1 was nocturia 0–1 ($n=60$), N2 was nocturia = 2 ($n=41$), and N3, ≥3 ($n=19$). Nocturia scores statistically decreased after RP in the N2 and N3 groups but worsened in the N1 group. It should also be noted that although a significant portion of the N2 and N3 groups improved, a majority of these patients never became free of nocturia and still complained of one to three episodes of nocturia following RP.

A follow-up study on the same patient population above noted that with longer follow-up after surgery (18 months), nocturia scores did not demonstrate the durable improvement over the time period as noted in other scores [27]. However, the N1 group discussed above did improve over time but never reached baseline levels. These RP studies suggest that nocturia is influenced markedly not only by obstruction of the prostatic urethra but also by bladder capacity/compliance, detrusor overactivity and sphincter weakness, or by increased production of urine at night [25–27]. Others have proposed that the wide anatomical dissection around the prostate during RP might disrupt the afferent and efferent innervations of the trigone and bladder neck to cause denervation of the bladder neck and detrusor muscle [26]. Decreased bladder compliance, detrusor overactivity, and increased voiding pressures have all been associated with this type of neural injury [28, 29].

Transurethral Resection of the Prostate

Trans urethral resection of the prostate (TURP) remains the gold standard therapy for LUTS related to BPH. TURP is the only transurethral procedure for BPH that has durable follow-up in the literature ranging from 8 to 22 years [30]. Ninety percent of patients report normal or improved voiding symptoms 10 years following therapy [31]. Madersbacher et al. [32] analyzed 29 randomized controlled trials comparing TURP to less-invasive procedures. The mean decrease in urinary symptom scores after TURP in the 29 studies was 70.6%. Symptom scores decreased by half in 58% of the patients. A meta-analysis compared urodynamic efficacy on various forms of bladder outlet obstruction therapies and found TURP to be better than all modalities except open prostatectomy [33]. It should be noted that most urodynamic measurements improve after surgery but they often do not correlate with LUTS as measured by symptom scores [34]. O'Sullivan et al. demonstrated that, in addition to improvement in AUA score, patients undergoing TURP had improvement in quality-of-life indices, depression rating scales, and pain indices at 1 month and 3 months postoperatively compared to baseline [35].

TURP for BPH has been associated with a 0.8–1.6 reduction in nocturia episodes per night [30, 31]. Multiple theories exist in why the surgery has its effect on nocturia. These include removal of the obstructing prostate tissue resulting in reinnervation of the bladder and subsequent resolution of detrusor overactivity [36]; destruction of the prostatic and bladder neck urothelium resulting in "deafferentation" of the afferent neurons responsible for initiating involuntary detrusor contractions [37, 38]; and the diminution in postvoid residual volume and subsequent increase in time for bladder filling [20].

Other Outlet Procedures

TURP procedures have decreased during the past decade secondary to competition from medical therapy for BPH and other minimally invasive surgical therapies (MIST) for BPH. These MIST therapies include: microwave ablation (TUMT); photoselective vaporization of the prostate (PVP laser); holmium laser enucleation of the prostate (HoLep); and transurethral vaporization of the prostate (TUVP). The total number of BPH procedures in Medicare patients increased 44% from 88,868 in 1999 to 127,786 in 2005 [39]. The number of MIST procedures for BPH increased 529% during this time frame [39]. Collaterally, by 2005 TURP encompassed only 39% of all BPH outlet procedures compared to 81% in 1999. A 2010 meta-analysis of all randomized controlled trials comparing MIST to TURP essentially demonstrated equivalent improvements in IPSS scores, peak flow rates and QOL indices among these procedures [40]. The strength of evidence of most randomized controlled trials comparing MIST to TURP has been questioned by multiple authors [41]. However, it is difficult to find analysis of TURP or MIST as it pertains specifically to improvement of nocturia. In fact, nocturia is not specifically addressed in most trials of outlet procedures: the metric focus of such trials is on postvoid residual volume change, perioperative complications and total IPSS.

Lee et al. specifically examined the effect of PVP laser on nocturia [30]. A total of 103 patients with BPH/LUTS who were refractory to medical therapy with at least two or more episodes of nocturia per night were evaluated prior to and following

80 W PVP laser therapy at intervals of 1, 3, 6, and 12 months postoperatively. Improvement of nocturia was defined as a reduction of over 50% in episodes. A statistically significant decrease in nocturia was noted starting from 1 month following PVP therapy. At 12 months following PVP, nocturnal frequency had decreased from a baseline mean of 3.0 ± 1.0 episodes to 2.1 ± 1.0 episodes. Preoperative nocturia or improvement of nocturia following PVP was not associated with the presence or absence of detrusor overactivity on urodynamic studies. The authors concluded that nocturia can improve significantly in the early postoperative period following PVP laser and proposed that the laser also destroys prostatic and bladder neck urothelium resulting in deafferentation much like a TURP.

Regression Analysis and NQOL with Outlet Procedures Related to Nocturia

Van Dijk et al. utilized logistic regression analysis to evaluate nocturia in 2,611 patients undergoing therapy for BPH/LUTS [4]. Four groups of patients that met inclusion criteria for BPH/LUTS were compared with regard to treatment effect. Patients were grouped into watchful waiting, alpha-blocker therapy, transurethral microwave thermotherapy (TUMT) and transurethral resection of the prostate (TURP). Age, prostate volume, and Q_{max} had small, statistically insignificant relation to treatment-associated improvements of nocturia. However, total IPSS score change had a significant contribution to nocturia improvement, reflecting the relatedness of nocturia with other items in the IPSS [4]. Regression analysis demonstrated watchful waiting and alpha-blocker therapy to have similar improvement on nocturia while TUMT and TURP were associated with a 0.3- and 0.6-point greater improvement in nocturia than alpha-blocker therapy. The authors also concluded through multivariate analysis that improvement in nocturia is more strongly associated with QOL improvement than is the case for other LUTS.

Cai et al. [3] utilized NQol in 61 men with BPH/LUTS to assess improvement following outlet surgery. Surgical treatment was associated with improvement of NQOL over a 6-month follow-up period. The type of surgical treatment elected had no effect on NQOL outcome. This study, however, did not look for predictors of NQOL improvement. A 2007 study utilized NQOL to assess improvement in nocturia following TURP ($n=36$) and simple prostatectomy ($n=20$) in patients with medically refractory BPH/LUTS [20]. NQOL was administered preoperatively and 2 or 3 months following surgery. NQOL scores increased from 24.1 ± 7 to 34.4 ± 7.5 following the outlet procedures. The outlet procedures also improved HUS from 1.83 ± 0.55 to 2.74 ± 0.64 during the follow-up period. Multivariate regression analysis demonstrated that HUS and the number of nocturia episodes per night were most predictive of NQOL score improvement. The improvement of HUS lead the investigators to conclude that a prostatectomy-induced reduction of even one nocturia event per night in men with LUTS/BPH may be clinically meaningful to improving quality of life.

Conclusions

Nocturia plays a significant role in quality of life and bother demonstrated in men with BPH/LUTS. Most studies evaluating surgical therapy for BPH fail to evaluate nocturia specifically except as a portion of reported IPSS questionnaires. Utilization of instruments more specific to nocturia and its effect on QOL such as the NQOL, and incorporation of regression analysis into studies evaluating outlet procedures, have allowed for insight into the impact of nocturia and its surgical therapy, on patient well-being. Studies utilizing NQOL as well as regression analysis suggest that surgery for BPH may improve nocturia more than previously thought and more rapidly than traditional studies suggest.

References

1. Kok ET, Schouten BW, Bohnen AM, Groeneveld FP, Thomas S, Bosch JL. Risk factors for lower urinary tract symptoms suggestive of benign prostatic hyperplasia in a community based population of healthy aging men: the Krimpen Study. J Urol. 2009;181:710–6.
2. Blanker MH, Bohnen AM, Groeneveld FPMJ, et al. Normal voiding patterns and determinants of increased diurnal and nocturnal voiding frequency in elderly men. J Urol. 2000;164:1201–5.
3. Cai T, Gardener N, Abraham L, Boddi V, Abrams P, Bartoletti R. Impact of surgical treatment on nocturia in men with benign prostatic obstruction. BJU Int. 2006;98:799–805.
4. van Dijk MM, Wijkstra H, Debruyne FM, de la Rosette JJMCH, Michel MC. The role of nocturia in the quality of life of men with lower urinary tract symptoms. BJU Int. 2009;105:1141–6.
5. Schneider T, de la Rosette JJMCH, Michel MC. Nocturia- a non-specific but important symptom of urologic disease. Int J Urol. 2009;16:249–56.
6. Chapple CR. Night time symptom control with Omnic (Tamsulosin) Oral Controlled Absorbtion System (OCAS). Eur Urol Suppl. 2005;4:14–6.
7. Barry M, Fowler F, O'Leary M, Bruskewitz R, Holtgrewe H, Mebust W. Measuring disease-specific health status in men with benign prostatic hyperplasia. Med Care. 1995;33:AS145–55.
8. Donovan JL. Measuring the impact of nocturia on quality of life. BJU Int. 1999;84 Suppl 1:21–5.
9. Asplund R. Mortality in the elderly in relation to nocturnal micturition. BJU Int. 1999;84:297–301.
10. Barry MJ, Fowler Jr FJ, O'Leary MP, et al. The American Urological Association symptom index for benign prostatic hyperplasia. The Measurement Committee of the American Urological Association. J Urol. 1992;148:1549–57.
11. Chancellor MB, Rivas DA. American Urological Association symptom index for women with voiding symptoms: lack of index specificity for benign prostatic hyperplasia. J Urol. 1993;150:1706–9.
12. Chancellor MB, Iivas DA, Keeley FX, et al. Similarity of the American Urologic Association symptom index among men with benign prostate hyperplasia (BPH), urethral obstruction not due to BPH and detrusor hyperreflexia without outlet obstruction. Br J Urol. 1994;74:200–3.
13. Madersbacher S, Pycha A, Klimgler CH, et al. The International Prostate Symptom score in both sexes: a urodynamics-based comparison. Neurourol Urodyn. 1999;18:173–82.
14. Barry MJ, Williford WO, Chang Y, et al. Benign prostatic hyperplasia specific health status measures in clinical research: how much change in the American Urological Association Symptom Index and the benign prostatic hyperplasia impact index is perceptible to patients? J Urol. 1995;154:1770–4.

15. Lepor H, Lowe FC. Chapter 39: Evaluation and nonsurgical management of benign prostatic hyperplasia. In: Walsh PC, Retik AB, Vaughan ED, Wein AJ, editors. Campbell's Urology. 8th ed. Philadelphia: Saunders Publishing; 2002.
16. Abraham L, Hareendran A, Mills IW, Martin ML, Abrams P, Drake MJ, et al. Development and validation of a quality-of-life measure for men with nocturia. Urology. 2004;63:481–6.
17. Guyatt GH, Feeny DH, Patrick DL. Measuring health-related quality of life. Ann Intern Med. 1993;118:622–9.
18. De Gennaro L, Martina M, Curcio G, Ferrara M. The relationship between alexithymia, depression, and sleep complaints. Psychiatry Res. 2004;128:253–8.
19. Johns MW. A new method for measuring daytime sleepiness: the Epworth sleepiness scale. Sleep. 1991;14:540–5.
20. Margel D, Lifshitz D, Brown N, Lask D, Pinhas LM, Tal R. Predictors of nocturia quality of life before and shortly after prostatectomy. Urology. 2007;70:493–7.
21. Mock LL, Parmalee PA, Kutner N, Scott J, Johnson TM. Content validation of symptom-specific nocturia quality-of-life instrument developed in men: Issues expressed by women, as well as men. Urology. 2008;72:736–42.
22. Akerstedt T, Nilsson PM. Sleep as restitution: an introduction. J Intern Med. 2003;254:6–12.
23. Chapple C, Batista JE, Berges R, et al. The impact of nocturia in patients with LUTS/BPH: need for new recommendations. Eur Urol Suppl. 2006;5:8–12.
24. Djavan B, Milani S, Davies J, et al. The impact of tamsulosin oral controlled absorption system (OCAS) on nocturia and the quality of sleep: preliminary results of a pilot study. Eur Urol Suppl. 2005;2:61–8.
25. Schwartz EJ, Lepor H. Radical retropubic prostatectomy reduces symptom scores and improves quality of life in men with moderate and severe lower urinary tract symptoms. J Urol. 1999;161:1185–8.
26. Namiki S, Saito S, Ishidoya S, Tochigi T, Ioritani N, Yoshimura K, et al. Adverse effect of radical prostatectomy on nocturia and voiding frequency symptoms. Urology. 2005;66:147–51.
27. Namiki S, Ishidoya S, Saito S, Satoh M, Tochigi T, Ioritani N, et al. Natural history of voiding function after radical retropubic prostatectomy. Urology. 2006;68:142–7.
28. Hellstrom P, Lukkarinen O, Kontturi M. Urodynamics in radical retropubic prostatectomy. Scan J Urol Nephrol. 1989;23:21–4.
29. Jung SY, Fraser MO, Ozawa H, et al. Urethral afferent nerve activity affects the micturition reflex: implication for the relationship between stress incontinence and detrusor instability. J Urol. 1999;162:204–12.
30. Reich O, Gratzke C, Stief CG. Techniques and long-term results of surgical procedures for BPH. Eur Urol. 2006;49:970–8.
31. Antunes AA, Srougi M, Coelho RF, Leite KR, Freire GC. Transurethral resection of the prostate for the treatment of lower urinary tract symptoms related to benign prostatic hyperplasia: How much should be resected. Int Bras J Urol. 2009;35(6):683–91.
32. Madersbacher S, Marberger M. Is transurethral resection of the prostate still justified? BJU Int. 1999;83:227–37.
33. Bosch JLHR. Urodynamic effects of various treatment modalities for benign prostatic hyperplasia. J Urol. 1997;158:2034–44.
34. Hakenberg OW, Pinnock CB, Marshall VR. Preoperative urodynamic and symptom evaluation of patients undergoing transurethral prostatectomy: analysis of variables relevant for outcome. BJU Int. 2003;91:375–9.
35. O'Sullivan MJ, Murphy C, Deasy C, Iohom G, Kiely EA, Shorten G. Effects of transurethral resection of prostate on the quality of life of patients with benign prostatic hyperplasia. J Am Coll Surg. 2004;198:394–403.
36. Cumming JA, Chisholm GD. Changes in detrusor innervations with relief of outflow tract obstruction. Br J Urol. 1992;69:7–11.
37. Lee CJ, Ch MC, Ku JH, Kim SW, Paick JS. Changes in nocturia after photoselective vaporization of the prostate for patients with benign prostatic hyperplasia. Korean J Urol. 2010;51:531–6.

38. Housami F, Abrams P. Persistent detrusor overactivity after transurethral resection of the prostate. Curr Urol Rep. 2008;9:284–90.
39. Yu X, Elliott SP, Wilt TJ, McBean AM. Practice patterns in benign prostatic hyperplasia surgical therapy: the dramatic increase in minimally invasive technologies. J Urol. 2008;180:241–5.
40. Ahyai SA, Gilling P, Kaplan SA, Kuntz RM, Madersbacher S, Montorsi F, et al. Meta-analysis of functional outcomes and complications following transurethral procedures for lower urinary tract symptoms resulting from benign prostatic enlargement. Eur Urol. 2010;58:384–97.
41. Burke N, Whelan JP, Goeree L, Hopkins RB, Campbell K, Goeree R, et al. Systematic review and meta-analysis of transurethral resection of the prostate versus minimally invasive procedures for the treatment of benign prostatic obstruction. Urology. 2010;75:1015–22.

Chapter 8
Lower Urinary Tract Pharmacotherapy for Nocturia

Roger Dmochowski and Alan J. Wein

Keywords Lower urinary tract pharmacotherapy • Nocturia • Antimuscarinic therapy • Overactive bladder • Management of obstructive BPH • Combined therapy • Antimuscarinics

Introduction

A variety of pharmacologic agents have been reported to have an effect on nocturia. Desmopressin is the agent most commonly specifically prescribed worldwide for nocturia related to nocturnal polyuria, and substantial evidence has been accrued using desmopressin for this indication. This chapter, however, focuses on reported results of treatment of nocturia with drugs directed toward the therapy of overactive bladder and lower urinary tract symptoms attributed to benign prostatic hyperplasia.

In considering the evidence for the benefits of pharmacologic treatment for nocturia, definitions for efficacy must be considered. Debate continues as to whether two or three episodes of awakenings due to the necessity to void is the threshold-significant nocturic frequency range. This debate, in part, focuses on the magnitude of symptomatic bother and associated reductions in quality of life, associated comorbidities, and the negative economic impact associated with nocturia. Therapeutic benefit thus should include a positive impact on the associated negative consequences of nocturia. Nonetheless, primary efficacy of therapy for nocturia should result in significant (statistical and clinical) decreases in nocturnal awakenings to void. However, extant evidence focuses almost solely on statistical reductions

R. Dmochowski, MD, FACS (✉)
Department of Urology, Vanderbilt University Medical Center, Nashville, TN, USA
e-mail: roger.dmochowski@vanderbilt.edu

A.J. Wein, MD, PhD (hon)
Department of Urology, University of Pennsylvania, Philadelphia, PA, USA

in nocturia episodes with no other corollary benefits (or lack thereof) reported. Recent consensus suggests that additional nonsubjective parameters such as increased time to first awakening, increased total daily sleep time, and changes in quality of life/comorbidities should be included in the overall therapeutic assessment of compounds being used for nocturia.

Nocturia Results with Antimuscarinic Therapy for Overactive Bladder

As nocturia is commonly seen in the overactive bladder symptom syndrome, and, when present at a frequency of two to three times or more, is one of the most bothersome of lower urinary tract symptoms, it is no great surprise that a common assumption is that these first line medications for overactive bladder exert a clinically significant effect on this symptom. Simple logic, however, would argue that this may not be so. Unless the antimuscarinics exert an effect on nocturnal polyuria, which they do not, they would be expected to exert an effect on nocturia only if the episodes of nocturia awakening were associated with urgency. A typical overactive bladder patient voids about 12 times during a 24-h period, and those who are bothered by nocturia complain of two to three such episodes at night, which are included in the 24 h frequency. Of the total voids in an overactive bladder patient, about 50% are associated with urgency, though the grade (severity) of urgency is variable. Thus, for every two voids, approximately one is associated with urgency. For a patient who has nocturia twice, this would mean one episode is due to urgency; for a patient with four nocturnal awakenings, two episodes are due to urgency; and for a patient with three nocturnal awakenings, 1.5 episodes are due to urgency. Antimuscarinics decrease urgency episodes by 50% at best, and the drug/placebo ratio is generally 2:1. This means that the best antimuscarinics could ever do, assuming this model is reasonably accurate, is to decrease, in a patient with "ordinary" overactive bladder, nocturia from 4 to 3, 3 to 2.25, or 2 to 1.5. Placebo would achieve approximately half the reduction, meaning the difference between drug and placebo would be 0.5, 0.375, and 0.25 episodes, respectively. Statistical considerations aside, and depending on the number of subjects in such a study, would the "man in the street" consider these reductions clinically significant? The only exception would be the group of patients with very severe urgency in whom the majority of their voids (counting urgency incontinence episodes as voids) were associated with urgency.

Brubaker and Fitzgerald [1] reported on the effect of solifenacin on male and female overactive bladder patients utilizing pooled data from four three-month phase III trials. As many as 2,534/3,032 patients who were randomized reported nocturia at baseline and 62% of the patients reporting nocturia were classified as having nocturnal polyuria. The baseline number of nocturic episodes was higher in those patients with nocturnal polyuria than those without (2.27–2.33 vs. 1.66–1.70). In those without nocturnal polyuria, there was a "significant" reduction in nocturia which amounted, however, to a numeric difference of 0.18 net advantage over placebo for the 5 mg dose and 0.08 for the 10 mg dose. For patients with nocturnal polyuria, the reductions were not significantly different from placebo (0.72 and 0.68 for the 5 and 10 mg doses, respectively, vs. 0.64 episodes for placebo). Cardozo et al. [2] reported on a double-blind placebo-controlled study which randomized 911/1091 patients to 5 or 10 mg of solifenacin and placebo for 12 weeks. The only statistically significant result was with 10 mg of drug which reduced nocturia from baseline by 0.71 episodes compared with placebo, which achieved 0.52 reduction. The reduction with the 5 mg dose was not significant. In the STAR study, a secondary analysis showed that both solifenacin and tolterodine were statistically effective in reducing nocturia episodes from baseline, but there was no placebo. The reduction and baseline for solifenacin were 0.71 and 2.02, and, for tolterodine, 0.63 and 1.92 [3]. Vardy et al. [4] reported on a double-blind placebo-controlled trial in patients flexibly dosed with solifenacin for 3 months. Solifenacin improved urgency incontinence and frequency, but not nocturia. The improvement with drug was 0.63 (baseline 1.7) and, for placebo, 0.48 (baseline 1.6).

Using trospium chloride, Rudy et al. (2006) [5] demonstrated a statistically significant decrease in the mean number of nocturic episodes per night (baseline 2) of 0.57 episodes for drug versus 0.29 episodes for placebo, a difference of 0.28 episodes. Zinner et al. (2004) [6] reported similar results with the same drug.

Johnson et al. (2005) [7] reported on a series of 131 women with nocturia who represented a subset of 197 with incontinence and urodynamic evidence of bladder dysfunction, defined as detrusor or a bladder capacity of <350 ml. Treatment arms were behavioral training (pelvic floor exercises); drug therapy (immediate release oxybutynin, dosage varying from 2.5 mg to 5 mg 3× daily); and placebo. Mean changes for the three groups were as follows: behavioral training, 1.9–1.4 episodes per night; drug therapy, 1.9 1.7; placebo, 1.9–2.0. The median change of 0.5 for behavioral training was statistically significantly better than drug (0.3) and placebo (0.0). Drug therapy was statistically better than placebo, but the clinical significance of this change is debatable. In the behavioral training group, 23.4% of patients experienced 50% less nocturia than at baseline as opposed to 8.7% for drug and 2.6% for placebo. Those who experienced a reduction of 1 full episode included 23.4% of behavioral training patients, 4.3% of drug-treated patients, and 7.9% of placebo-treated patients.

There has been a group of studies done with tolterodine and with the newer agent, fesoterodine, which seem to reflect the spectrum of results seen with older antimuscarinic agents. Rackley et al. (2006) [8] reported on the median percentage reduction in nocturnal micturition frequency with tolterodine, dividing the nocturnal voids into nonoveractive bladder voids, OAB voids, and severe OAB voids, – those associated with severe urgency on an urgency scale described in the manuscript. Overall, there was no significant effect over placebo on nocturia episodes, a finding also reported by Nitti et al. (2006) [9]. However, with nighttime dosing, there was a statistically significant improvement in OAB-related nocturnal voids (those associated with urgency). The percentage change in OAB associated nocturia was −30 for drug and −22 for placebo. For "severe" OAB-associated nocturia, the percent reductions were 59 for drug and 43 for placebo, also statistically significant. These results

Table 8.1 Collected results of recent studies with data for effect of fesoterodine on nocturia

	Median% decrease	Mean#↓/baseline
Chapple et al. [12]		
Placebo	27	0.32/1.8
Tolt ER 4 mg	25 NS	0.40/2.0 NS
Feso 4 mg	29 NS	0.39/1.9 NS
Feso 8 mg	24 NS	0.39/2.0 NS
Nitti et al. [13]		
Placebo	25	0.39/2.0
Feso 4 mg	33 p 0.13	0.58/2.2 p 0.42
Feso 8 mg	25 NS	0.55/1.9 p 0.09
Herschorn et al. [14]		
Placebo	25	0.5/2.3
Tolt ER 4 mg	28 NS	0.6/2.2 NS
Feso 8 mg	29 NS	0.6/2.2 NS
Dmochowski et al. [15]		
Placebo	No difference in mean nocturnal voids or	?/2.7
Feso (Titrated 4–8 mg)	nocturnal urgency episodes for either	?/2.6

were maintained in a study of men with overactive bladder – dry [10, 11]. However, when one looks at the absolute reductions in the Rackley et al. (2006) [8] study, one realizes that it is hard to argue clinical significance, even in the statistically significant groups. The baseline OAB nocturnal voids for drug and placebo were 2.5 and 2.4. Calculating the absolute reduction from the percentage reductions, it is hard to argue that the differences would have been clinically noticeable. However, these results do argue for proof of concept with respect to reduction in urgency episodes with antimuscarinic agents and, further, suggest that antimuscarinics potentially offer the most benefit to patients with significant and severe frequent urgency without nocturnal polyuria, an opinion shared by Brubaker and Fitzgerald (2007) [1].

Chapple et al. (2007) [12], Nitti et al. (2007) [13], and Herschorn et al. (2010) [14] all carried out studies looking at the effects of fesoterodine on nocturia, some looking also at a comparison of this with extended release tolterodine (4 mg). The results for median percent decreases in nocturia, the mean absolute decrease in nocturia, and the baseline nocturia are seen in Table 8.1. None show any clinical significance. Dmochowski et al. (2010) [15] reported on a dose titration study of fesoterodine versus placebo. The nocturia baselines were 2.7 for placebo and 2.6 for drug. There were no significant changes for either nocturia or nocturnal urgency episodes.

Therapies Used for the Management of Obstructive BPH

Several assessments of drugs used primarily for bladder outlet obstruction secondary to benign enlargement of the prostate have included an assessment of drug effect on nocturic frequency. Many of the studies show benefits with alpha-blockers;

however, either no other outcomes are reported or methodological considerations exist. Roehrborn et al. (2003) [16], comparing alfuzosin to placebo, showed a net change in nocturic episodes over placebo of 0.3 voids per night, which was statistically significant. No other outcomes related to nocturia were reported. Koseoglu et al. (2006) [17] found that nocturnal polyuria in up to 95% of patients with LUTS suggestive of BPO produced resistance to $alpha_1$ blockade therapy. Despite this, 20 men (mean nocturia 3.3 episodes) treated with tamsulosin for 6 weeks (no placebo) experienced a statistically significant reduction to 2.4 nocturic episodes per night. Vallancien et al. (2008) [18] noted a reduction of 0.8 voids per night utilizing alfuzosin (post hoc analysis of a 3-year uncontrolled open-label study in 689 patients with bladder outlet obstructive symptoms). Ukimura et al. (2008) [19] evaluated a small patient sample with "marked nighttime polyuria" excluded, comparing naftopidil and tamsulosin after 6 weeks of therapy. Nocturia, as calculated from the IPSS nocturia score, decreased from 3.5 to 1.6 episodes with naftopidil, and from 3.4 to 1.7 with tamsulosin. Although statistically significant over baseline, such studies generally amount to "usage studies" (Wein and Dmochowski 2007) [20], and their clinical significance is in question.

Johnson et al. (2003) [21] reported a secondary analysis of the Veterans' Administration Cooperative Study using IPSS-derived nocturia data. The study included four treatment groups: terazosin, finasteride, combination terazosin plus finasteride, and placebo. The authors assessed 1,078 men, age 45–80, with a diagnosis of "BPH" followed for 1 year for reductions in nocturia. At baseline, 96.5% of patients had nocturia at least once and 75.8% had nocturia at least twice. Overall changes in nocturia events at study end included: placebo reduction from 2.4 to 2.1, terazosin reduction, 2.4 to 1.8, finasteride reduction, 2.5 to 2.1, and combination reduction, 2.4 to 2.0, with only the terazosin arm being statistically significantly from the other arms. Combination therapy was statistically significantly different from finasteride and placebo. The study defined a 50% reduction in nocturia as being meaningful; however, only a 17% greater improvement for alpha-blocker over placebo for nocturia was seen. The authors concluded that effects on nocturia "correlated with changes in the reported bother from nocturia," and they termed the effect "moderate" on "symptom specific quality of life measures."

Speakman (2006) [22] evaluated tamsulosin OCAS 0.4 mg in men with LUTS/BPH and 2 or more nocturnal voids, from a secondary evaluation of results initially reported by Djavan et al. (2005) [23]. Tamsulosin OCAS 0.4 mg was found to be (slightly) superior to placebo in reducing nocturia as captured by the IPSS, with changes of 3.1–2.3 for placebo and 3.1–2.0 for drug. No significant difference in the time to the first awakening to void was noted.

Data from the MTOPS trial were analyzed by Johnson et al. (2007) [24]. The study included four groups: doxazosin alone, finasteride alone, combination, and placebo. At 1- and 4-year follow-up, change in self-reported nocturia from baseline was reported. Mean nocturia episodes at baseline were 2.3, 2.4, 2.3, 2.3, respectively. After 1 year of therapy, mean reduction in nocturia were: doxazosin, 0.45; finasteride, 0.4; doxazosin and finasteride (combination), 0.58; placebo, 0.35. After 4 years of treatment, reductions were similar (0.53, 0.42, 0.55, 0.38). In men with two or more nocturia episodes at baseline, episode reductions (at 1 and 4 years) were: doxazosin, 0.77 and 0.77, finasteride, 0.60 and 0.68, combination, 0.80 and 0.79, and placebo, 0.61 and 0.66. At 4 years of follow-up, only doxazosin versus placebo reductions reached significance. When re-evaluated for two or more episodes at baseline, significant reductions were noted for both doxazosin and combination therapy versus placebo and versus finasteride at 1 year. The overall magnitude of difference between the active arms and placebo, although statistically significant in some circumstances, do not appear to have clinical significance.

Combined Therapy

The results of the two analyses by Johnson et al. (2003, 2007) [21, 24] that looked at combination therapy (an alpha-blocker and a 5 alpha-reductase inhibitor) have been discussed previously. Kaplan et al. (2006) [10, 11] reported on a combination of tamsulosin and extended release tolterodine for the treatment of men with lower urinary tract symptoms and overactive bladder in a four-arm, 12-week study. The change in micturitions at night from baseline was significant only for the combination group, amounting to a decrease of 0.6 episodes per night (baseline 2.07), with a change in placebo, however, of nearly 0.4 (baseline 2.02). Vaughn et al. (2009) [25] looked at multimodal treatment in a pilot study of a small number of men, mean age 67 (51–85), all of whom had nocturia at least two times. All subjects received behavioral modification. Those characterized as having BPH received terazosin, titrated to 10 mg. Those with daily frequency eight or more times received tolterodine (2 mg immediate release twice daily or extended release 4 mg once daily). Men who required more than 30 min to return to sleep received zaleplon 5 mg (a non-benzodiazepine sedative/hypnotic). Seventy-five percent of the patients studied received one drug, 20% two drugs, and 5% no drugs. There were no intra-group comparisons. There was no placebo arm. On a bladder diary, the mean nocturia episode change was 3.1–1.1, and on an AUA symptom score tabulation, 2.6–1.1.

Other Studies

Addla et al. (2006) [26] reported on the use of a nonsteroidal anti-inflammatory drug, diclofenac, for patients with nocturnal polyuria. This was a small study, 26 patients, but was placebo controlled with a crossover. The mean nocturnal frequency statistically decreased, but numerically improved only from 2.8 to 2.3 episodes per night. The placebo effect was much lower than that generally seen, 2.8–2.7 episodes per night, perhaps owing to the pathophysiology. Nine patients or 34.6% improved greater than 0.5 episodes on drug. In a somewhat unusual study, Kaye et al. (2008) [27] published the results of a self-study which was blinded. The agents utilized were placebo, oxazepam (a short acting benzodiazepine), naproxen (an NSAID), zopiclone (a non-benzodiazepine sedative), oxycodone (an opioid), trazadone (an SNRI sedative/antidepressant), and placebo. Each medication, blinded by a pharmacist, was taken 10 times for a total of 60 tests. The mean number of nocturia episodes for placebo was 1.6. Statistically significant differences were achieved with oxazepam (0.6 episodes per night) and naproxen (0.7). Out of a possible 10, four nocturia-free nights were achieved with oxazepam and five with naproxen. Detailed metabolic records were kept and it was noted that oxazepam produced no change in urine volume while naproxen reduced water, salt, and potassium excretion, reducing the volume of urine by 46%.

In summary, there has been little success in the treatment of nocturia with 5-ARI agents given to patients for relief of symptoms due to bladder outlet obstruction caused by prostatic enlargement. There have been occasional placebo-controlled reports of statistically significant, but in our opinion not clinically significant, decreases with alpha adrenergic blockade therapy, and the same can be said for combination therapy with these two types of agents. Statistical success has been achieved in some groups with a variety of antimuscarinic agents, but in our opinion, the clinical significance of these changes in the groups studied is doubtful. Hypothetically, one would have to select a group of patients with a large number of nocturia episodes, most of which were due to detrusor overactivity-related urgency, to potentially see a clinically significant result. It is also likely, however, that these agents will continue to play a role in reducing symptoms of patients with LUTS attributable to bladder outlet obstruction and to overactive bladder. However, it is also likely that other types of therapies, perhaps in combination, will need to be employed in order to achieve a clinically significant reduction in nocturia.

References

1. Brubaker L, Fitzgerald MP. Nocturnal polyuria and nocturia relief in patients treated with solifenacin for overactive bladder symptoms. Int Urogynecol J. 2007;18:737–41.
2. Cardozo L, Lisec M, Millard R, Trip VAN Vierssen O, Kuzmin I, Drogendijk TE, et al. Randomized, double- blind placebo controlled trial of the once daily antimuscarinic agent solifenacin succinate in patients with overactive bladder. J Urol. 2004;172:1919–24.
3. Chapple CR, Martinez-Garcia R, Selvaggi L, Toozs-Hobson P, Warnack W, Drogendiji T, et al. A comparison of the efficacy and tolerability of solifenacin succinate and extended release tolterodine at treating overactive bladder syndrome: results of the STAR trial. Eur Urol. 2005;48:464–70.
4. Vardy MD, Mitcheson HD, Samuels T-A, Wegenke JD, Forero-Schwanhaeuser S, Marshall TS, et al. Effects of solifenacin on overactive bladder symptoms, symptom bother and other patient-reported outcomes: results from VIBRANT – a double-blind, placebo-controlled trial. Int J Clin Pract. 2009;63(12):1702–14.
5. Rudy D, Cline K, Harris R, Goldberg K, Dmochowski R. Multicenter phase III trial studying trospium chloride in patients with overactive bladder. Urology. 2006;67:275–80.
6. Zinner N, Gittelman M, Harris R, Susset J, Kanellos A, Auerbach S. Trospium chloride improves overactive bladder symptoms: a multicenter phase III trial. J Urol. 2004;171:2311–5.
7. Johnson-II TM, Burgio KL, Redden DT, Wright KC, Goode PS. Effects of behavioral and drug therapy on nocturia in older incontinent women. J Am Geriatr Soc. 2005;53(5):846–50.

8. Rackley R, Weiss JP, Rovner ES, Wang JT, Guan Z. Nighttime dosing with tolterodine reduces bladder-related nocturnal micturitions in patients with overactive bladder and nocturia. Urology. 2006;67:731–6.
9. Nitti VW, Dmochowski R, Appell RA, Wang JT, Bavendam T, Guan Z. Efficacy and tolerability of tolterodine extended-release in continent patients with overactive bladder and nocturia. BJU Int. 2006;97:1262–6.
10. Kaplan SA, Roehrborn CG, Rovner ES, Carlsson M, Bavendam T, Guan Z. Tolterodine and Tamsulosin for treatment of men with lower urinary tract symptoms and overactive bladder. A randomized controlled trial. JAMA. 2006;296:2319–28.
11. Kaplan SA, Roehrborn CG, Dmochowski R, Rovner ER, Wang JT, Guan Z. Tolterodine extended release improves overactive bladder symptoms in men with overactive bladder and nocturia. Urology. 2006;68(2):328–32.
12. Chapple C, Van Kerrebroeck P, Tubaro A, Haag-Molkenteller C, Forst H-T, Massow U, et al. Clinical efficacy, safety and tolerability of once-daily fesoterodine in subjects with overactive bladder. Eur Urol. 2007;52:1204–12.
13. Nitti VW, Dmochowski R, Sand PK, Forst H-T, Haag-Molkenteller C, Massow U, et al. Efficacy and tolerability of fesoterodine for overactive bladder syndrome. J Urol. 2007;178:2488–94.
14. Herschorn S, Swift S, Guan Z, Carlsson M, Morrow JD, Brodsky M, et al. Comparison of fesoterodine and tolterodine extended release for the treatment of overactive bladder: a head-to-head placebo controlled trial. BJU Int. 2010;105:58–66.
15. Dmochowski RR, Peters KM, Morrow JD, Guan Z, Gong J, Sun F, et al. Randomized, double-blind, placebo controlled trial of flexible-dose fesoterodine in subjects with overactive bladder. Urology. 2010;75:62–8.
16. Roehrborn CG, Van Kerrebroeck P, Nordling J. Safety and efficacy of alfuzosin 10 mg once-daily in the treatment of lower urinary tract symptoms and clinical benign prostatic hyperplasia: a pooled analysis of three double-blind, placebo-controlled studies. BJU Int. 2003;92:257–61.
17. Koseoglu H, Aslan G, Ozdemir I, Esen A. Nocturnal polyuria in patients with lower urinary tract symptoms and response to alpha blocker therapy. Urology. 2006;67:1188–92.
18. Vallancien G, Emberton M, Alcaraz A, Matzkin H, van Moorselaar RJA, Hartung R, et al. Alfuzosin 10mg once daily for treating benign prostatic hyperplasia: a 3-year experience in real life practice. BJU Int. 2008;101:847–52.
19. Ukimura O, Kanazawa M, Fujihara A, et al. Naftopidil versus tamsulosin hydrochloride for lower urinary tract symptoms associated with benign prostatic hyperplasia with special reference to the storage symptom: a prospective randomized controlled study. Int J Urol. 2008;15:1049–54.
20. Wein A, Dmochowski R. Strategies for data comparison for drugs used in the treatment of overactive bladder. In: Kreder K, Dmochowski R, editors. The overactive bladder, evaluation and management. London: Informa Healthcare; 2007. p. 239–52.
21. Johnson-II TM, Jones K, Williford WO, Kutner MH, Issa MM, Lepor H. Changes in nocturia from medical treatment of benign prostatic hyperplasia: secondary analysis of the department of veterans affairs cooperative study trial. J Urol. 2003;170:145–8.
22. Speakman M. Efficacy and safety of tamsulosin OCAS. BJU Int. 2006;98 suppl 2:13–7.
23. Djavan B, Milani S, Davies J, Boledoeoku J. The impact of tamsulosin oral controlled absorption system on nocturia and the quality of sleep: preliminary results of a pilot study. Eur Urol. 2005;4(suppl):61–8.
24. Johnson-II TM, Burrows PK, Kusek JW, Nyberg LM, Tenover JL, Lepor H, et al. The effect of doxazosin, finasteride and combination therapy on nocturia in men with benign prostatic hyperplasia. J Urol. 2007;178:2045–51.
25. Vaughn CP, Endeshaw Y, Nagamia Z, Ouslander JG, Johnson TM. A multicomponent behavioural and drug intervention for nocturia in elderly men: rationale and pilot results. BJU Int. 2009;104:69–74.
26. Addla SK, Adeyoju AB, Neilson D, O'Reilly P. Diclofenac for treatment of nocturnal polyuria: a prospective, randomised, double-blind, placebo-controlled crossover study. Eur Urol. 2006;49:720–6.
27. Kaye M. Nocturia: a blinded, randomized, parallel placebo-controlled self-study of the effect of 5 different sedatives and analgesics. Can Urol Assoc J. 2008;2(6):604–8.

Chapter 9
Nocturia and Antidiuretic Pharmacotherapy

Philip E.V. Van Kerrebroeck

Keywords Antidiuretic Pharmacotherapy • Arginine vasopressin (AVP) • Desmopressin • Hyponatremia • Nocturia • Overactive Bladder (OAB) • The Noctopus trials

Introduction

Sleep loss caused by the frequent need to void at night inflicts a heavy burden on patients with nocturia and their partners. Nocturia is defined as the need to wake one or more times at night to void, with each void preceded and followed by sleep [1], but studies of the relationship between QoL (quality of life) and nocturia suggest that nocturia becomes clinically significant when ≥2 voids per night are experienced [2, 3]. At this level, nocturia is consistently found to be one of the most troublesome lower urinary tract symptoms (LUTS) [4, 5], significantly compromising sleep and overall QoL [6, 7]. Many people consider nocturia to be one of the inevitable consequences of growing old despite, or perhaps because of, the fact that it is highly prevalent, affecting approximately half of the adult population, and increasing with age [8]. However, the condition also affects a significant proportion of younger adults [9], and the QoL and sleep-related consequences can have a serious impact on the lives of patients and their partners [10, 11]. If patients are bothered by the condition, it would seem to be appropriate to investigate and address the specific causes contributing to nocturnal voiding frequency.

Because multiple behavioral, physiological, and pathological factors may cause nocturia, the latter is still not well understood in clinical practice, leading to partial or inaccurate diagnosis and, in many cases, inadequate treatment [12]. Common

P.E.V. Van Kerrebroeck, MD, PhD, MMSc (✉)
Department of Urology, University Hospital Maastricht, Maastricht, The Netherlands
e-mail: urolmaas@hotmail.com

urological causes of nocturia have been classified into four broad categories: 24-h polyuria (excessive urine production during the day and night), bladder storage problems (e.g., overactive bladder, OAB, and BPH), nocturnal polyuria (NP) or significant overproduction of urine at night, and mixed etiology (e.g., OAB+NP) [12]. The NP category is perhaps the largest, but these patients are also the most likely to receive an incomplete diagnosis and fail to respond to first-line treatment intended to address only one underlying factor.

Nocturia has been traditionally regarded by urologists as a storage symptom associated with benign prostatic problems (BPH) and/or OAB [13, 14], and treatments have been primarily directed at either reducing bladder overactivity or removing BOO, sometimes surgically. However, such therapeutic approaches have proven to be ineffective against nocturia in many studies of OAB and BPH therapy [14–16]. A likely explanation for this is suggested by data showing that NP (defined as an age-dependent nocturnal urine volume >20–33% of the 24-h urine volume) has an extremely high prevalence in patients with nocturia (up to 82.9%) and is the single-most common cause of the condition in urological patients (see Chapters 7 and 8) [13, 17]. If NP is present (alone or with other factors) but not diagnosed or treated, nocturia will persist. Indeed, in a study of patients with an OAB diagnosis receiving the anticholinergic solifenacin, only patients without NP showed significant improvement in their nocturia episodes [14]. Even among those without NP, the decrease in nocturnal voiding was only marginally better than with placebo (0.18 fewer episodes per night). Similarly, in a study of nocturia patients with BPH receiving α-blocker therapy, treatment for BPH did not improve nocturia symptoms and further analysis revealed that 95% of patients had NP in addition to BPH [15]. Furthermore, prostate surgery is reported to have modest effect on nocturia [18]. These studies highlight the importance of greater recognition of NP among clinicians, so they can offer improved diagnosis and treatment options to patients with nocturia.

NP is itself a multifactorial condition. The cause in some patients may be as simple as excessive fluid intake before bedtime. However, if the condition is not remedied by modifying drinking behaviors, other etiologies may be suspected. A key contributor is a blunting of the normal circadian rhythm of antidiuretic hormone (arginine vasopressin) release. Other issues suggested to be related to NP, but which have varying levels of evidence, include hypertension, renal insufficiency, congestive heart failure, cardiovascular conditions, or sleep apnea [19]. Based on these findings, it is logical to aim at antidiuretic therapy as a major therapeutic modality in the majority of patients with significant nocturia after conservative measures failed.

Antidiuretic Pharmacotherapy

For patients whose nocturia is related to nocturnal polyuria, either alone or in combination with OAB or BPH, treatment that reduces nocturnal urine volumes may be warranted [20].

The antidiuretic hormone arginine vasopressin (AVP) plays a key role in the control of urine production. Hence, the manipulation of AVP presents an opportunity for therapeutic use. To date, desmopressin, a synthetic analog of AVP, is the only available antidiuretic drug and has been used for over 30 years in the treatment of disorders such as diabetes insipidus (DI) and primary nocturnal enuresis (PNE). More recently, it has been introduced for the treatment of nocturia with a polyuric background.

Assuming that patients have been given advice regarding night-time fluid intake, and other causes of NP have been excluded, then antidiuretic therapy may be an appropriate choice since it can address insufficient secretion of arginine vasopressin, which results in NP and, frequently, nocturia.

Antidiuretic therapy with the synthetic analog of AVP, desmopressin, is the only pharmacological therapy which in many countries is indicated specifically for nocturia. Desmopressin is a selective V_2 receptor agonist and therefore has a greater specificity of action than AVP, avoiding unwanted vasopressor and uterotonic effects associated with V_1 agonism [21]. Desmopressin has a more powerful and longer-lasting antidiuretic action than AVP. It increases reabsorption of water in the distal and collecting tubules of the kidney via its action on the V_2 receptor, and concentrates the urine, decreasing urine production, and postponing the need to void.

Given the specific antidiuretic action of desmopressin, it is the pharmacological therapy of choice for patients with nocturia where NP is present, and has a grade A level 1 recommendation from the International Consultation on Incontinence [22]. It has a fast onset of action, with urine production decreasing within 30 min of oral administration [23] and can be administered as a tablet or oral lyophilisate ("melt") formulation requiring no concomitant fluid intake. The oral lyophilisate formulation has greater bioavailability than the tablet, allowing lower dosing to achieve equivalent antidiuresis and a well-defined duration of action with different dosages in children suffering from bedwetting [24].

Structure and Mechanism of Action of Desmopressin

The antidiuretic hormone arginine vasopressin (AVP) plays a key role in the control of urine production and hence the manipulation of AVP presents an opportunity for therapeutic use. To date, desmopressin, a synthetic analog of AVP, is the only available antidiuretic drug, and has been used for over 30 years in the treatment of disorders such as diabetes insipidus (DI) and primary nocturnal enuresis (PNE). More recently, it has been introduced for the treatment of nocturia with a polyuric background. Furthermore, several studies have indicated that antidiuretic treatment is effective in patients with urinary incontinence and/or OAB. Although desmopressin is a well-established antidiuretic treatment, new indications for the drug are still being evaluated.

Desmopressin is a synthetic analog of the body's own antidiuretic hormone, AVP. Desmopressin is a nonapeptide with two cysteine residues, forming a bridge between positions 1 and 6. The omission of the amino group in position 1 and the introduction of a D-enantiomer in place of L-arginine at position 8 make desmopressin

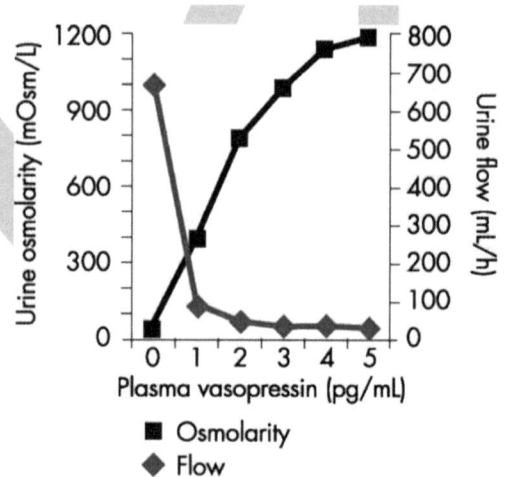

Fig. 9.1 The relation between plasma vasopressin, urine osmolality, and urine flow (figure adapted from Robertson and Norgaard [27])

more potent, stable, and long acting than AVP. Unlike AVP, desmopressin is V_2-receptor specific and therefore has a greater specificity of action than AVP. As a consequence, it reduces urine production without inducing unwanted vasopressor and uterotonic effects associated with V_1 agonism [25, 26].

Desmopressin has a more powerful and longer-lasting antidiuretic action than AVP. It increases reabsorption of water in the distal and collecting tubules of the kidney via its action on the V_2 receptor, and concentrates the urine, decreasing urine production and postponing the need to void (Fig. 9.1) [27].

Trials with Desmopressin

Two sets of trials, the European Noctopus trials and the USA–Canada Melt trial, evaluated the clinical effects of the treatment with desmopressin for nocturia.

The Noctopus Trials

The Noctopus trials were a program of three short-term, randomized, double-blind, placebo-controlled, multicenter, phase III trials carried out in men and women with nocturia. The Noctopus trials were primarily conducted in Europe. These studies investigated the safety and efficacy of desmopressin tablets in the treatment of nocturia. The studies shared a similar study design and inclusion/exclusion criteria. Data on NP status were collected during screening via 7-day FVCs in which subjects recorded urine volume, fluid intake, and frequency of micturition. NP was defined as a nocturnal urine volume >33% of the 24-h urine voided, including the first morning void.

Subjects ≥18 years of age reporting ≥2 voids per night were screened. Exclusion criteria were adopted to ensure that nocturia was not due to well-defined causes of increased urinary frequency which require specific management, such as multiple sclerosis, diabetes insipidus, or polydipsia. Subjects were excluded due to pregnancy, hematuria, bacteriuria, pyuria, proteinuria, glucosuria or ketonuria, low serum sodium, treatment within 30 days of study start with drugs known or suspected to interact with desmopressin, BPH medical/surgical treatment initiated <6 months earlier, uncontrolled hypertension, clinically relevant cardiac failure, renal or hepatic disease, known alcohol or drug abuse, other investigational drugs taken in the past 30 days, any history of clinically relevant psychiatric disorders within the 24 months preceding enrollment in the trial, and work or lifestyle factors potentially interfering with regular night-time sleep (e.g., shift workers). However, information on whether patients excluded from entry to the Noctopus trials were eliminated from the sample prior to or following completion of the baseline FVCs is not available; therefore, it is possible that the cohort included in the current study of FVC data may include a small number of patients with the above conditions.

A total of 1,003 patients (519 males, 484 females) were screened for the three studies [20–22]. In the total population 157/1,003 (16%) were non-evaluable due to incomplete FVCs.

The prevalence of NP in patients with evaluable records was 76% (641/846). If patients with non-valuable records were assumed to be nonpolyurics, the proportion with NP was 64% (641/1,003).

The frequency of NP increased significantly with age. The frequency of NP in those <65 years was 66% (325/493), and 90% in those ≥65 years (316/353) (Chi-square test, $p<0.0001$). A breakdown of the screened population by sex revealed that the prevalence of NP was significantly higher in males (79%; 352/446) than in females (72%; 289/400) (Chi-square test, $p=0.02$). Rates of NP were high in all ethnic groups (≥63%). However, in these studies, small numbers of subjects in the Asian and Hispanic groups were represented.

In the short-term (3 weeks) trials, 33% of male and 46% of female desmopressin treated patients showed a >50% reduction in the mean number of voids per night relative to baseline ($p<0.001$ and $p<0.0001$, respectively, compared with placebo). All other efficacy endpoints, including the mean number of nocturnal voids and the duration of the first sleep period until the first nocturnal void, showed a highly significant difference in favor of desmopressin compared with placebo(64,65). QoL analyses also indicated a greater improvement in terms of prevalence, bother, and problems caused by nocturia, in patients treated with desmopressin compared with placebo.

Of patients completing the short-term Noctopus studies, 88% entered the 10–12-month extension study. At 12 months, the proportion of patients with a >50% reduction in the number of nocturnal voids compared with baseline increased from 37 to 67% in males, and from 46 to 67% in females. Overall, efficacy in all endpoints and the improvement in QoL were maintained during long-term treatment.

Short- and long-term studies show that desmopressin is well tolerated, with a low incidence of adverse events that are comparable with the established safety profile of the drug in other indications.

Inappropriate water intake that can lead to hyponatremia is the main safety consideration. Pooled analysis of the Noctopus trials showed that the risk of hyponatremia increases with age, with the over-65-year group at most risk. Therefore, the initiation of treatment in this age group is not recommended, unless under close supervision.

Desmopressin has also been shown to alleviate nocturia due to nocturnal polyuria in patients with Parkinson's disease [28]. It may also be effective in the treatment of nocturia not associated with nocturnal polyuria, for example, in patients with benign prostatic enlargement [29], neurogenic bladder due to multiple sclerosis [30–33] and detrusor over activity refractory to evening fluid restriction and antispasmodic therapy [34]. It has been given a level 1, grade A recommendation by the International Consultation on Incontinence for the treatment of nocturia [35].

These data show that NP is a major contributing factor to nocturia, with a prevalence of 76% in patients screened for clinical trials who provided evaluable diary data. Additionally, the data indicate that although the prevalence of NP increased with age, it was present in the majority of subjects both under and over 65 years of age (66–83% of <65 years and 90–93% of ≥65 years). The high prevalence of NP found in all trials and all subgroups suggests that this is a leading cause of nocturia in men and women of all ages.

In these trials, ≥64% of subjects had NP, if those without evaluable data were assumed not to have NP. These findings are consistent with previous reports in the literature regarding the high prevalence of NP in patients with nocturia [13–15, 36], and the suboptimal results of treating nocturia with traditional OAB and BPH therapies [37, 38].

The potential for inadequate diagnosis in patients with NP is twofold: first, some patients may be wrongly diagnosed with OAB or BPH because this is the traditional assumption for patients with LUTS; second, some patients may indeed have OAB or BPH, but in combination with NP. The danger for these patients is that NP will go undetected, since clinicians may be more comfortable with the (also accurate) OAB or BPH diagnosis. This therefore has a major impact on nocturia therapy, indicating a need to consider this condition – which can have serious consequences for the health and well-being of patients – as a distinct clinical entity, often with a multifactorial pathogenesis, and sometimes independent from other LUTS. Following exclusion of other major conditions such as neurogenic disorders, nocturia deserves full evaluation using an FVC to ascertain whether 24-h voiding volumes are excessive (24-h polyuria), or volumes are excessive only at night (NP), or there are small voided volumes (bladder storage problems), or whether a combination of these factors is present. Treatment offered should be directed toward the specific cause(s) identified in each patient to increase the likelihood of achieving a clinically meaningful reduction in nocturia.

Nocturia is often assumed to indicate bladder dysfunction or BOO. However, this study and others demonstrate that NP, an overproduction of urine at night, is present in the overwhelming majority of patients with nocturia, including those with persistent nocturia despite BPH and OAB therapy. This finding is consistent regardless of sex, age, and ethnicity. Evaluation and treatment of patients with nocturia should therefore give full consideration to the multifactorial etiology of the condition, and to the possibility that there may be more than one causal factor which needs to be addressed.

USA and Canada Trial

The second source of information on the role of desmopressin in nocturia treatment is a recent large, randomized, double-blind, placebo-controlled, phase III clinical trial in the USA and Canada. This study investigated the effects of a new fast-dissolving formulation of desmopressin (oral lyophilisate/melt) in the treatment of nocturia (USA and Canada Trial) [39].

This was a large randomized, double-blind, placebo-controlled, phase III trial carried out in a broad population of men and women with nocturia, recruited from 81 sites in the USA and Canada. Data on NP status were collected during screening at baseline via 3-day FVCs; patients were instructed to record the time and volume of each void for three consecutive 24-h periods (daytime and nighttime). The nocturnal urine volume included the volume of the first morning void. Patients were instructed to empty their bladder before going to bed and to limit fluid intake to satisfy thirst only; evening intake of liquids with diuretic effect was especially discouraged.

Men and women ≥18 years reporting an average of ≥2 voids per night were included. Patients with BPH or OAB were included if they had been diagnosed and adequately treated prior to screening. Patients were excluded if they showed any of the following conditions: congestive heart failure, uncontrolled hypertension, uncontrolled diabetes mellitus, renal insufficiency, hepatic/biliary disease, current or past urologic malignancy, active urinary tract pathology, severe pelvic prolapse, neurogenic detrusor overactivity, diabetes insipidus, polydipsia, hyponatremia at baseline, syndrome of inappropriate antidiuretic hormone secretion, obstructive sleep apnea requiring therapy, or any surgical procedure <6 months prior to screening. If on any of the following pharmacological therapies, subjects must have been on a stable dose for >3 months prior to screening: α-blockers, 5α-reductase inhibitors, antispasmodics, anticholinergics or antimuscarinics for OAB, sedative/hypnotic medications for sleep disorders, selective serotonin and mixed norepinephrine/serotonin reuptake inhibitors, chronic use of non-steroidal anti-inflammatory agents, diabinese, carbamazepine and amiodarone.

Of 1,412 subjects screened for this study (767 males, 644 females; data on sex missing for one screened subject), 917 (65%) were eligible and completed a 3-day FVC during the screening procedure.

The prevalence of NP in patients who completed the FVCs during the screening phase was 88% (806/917). If we assume that all those who did not fill in the diary did not have NP, the most conservative estimate of NP prevalence is ≥57% (806/1,412) of all screened patients.

Of the screened population, 43% (613/1412) were excluded from the phase III study. The most common reasons for screening failure were renal insufficiency

(15%), not averaging ≥2 nocturnal voids over the 3-day screening period (10%) and hyponatremia (4%).

Of the 799 randomized subjects, 89% (711/799) had NP. Two females and one male had unknown NP status.

The frequency of NP in the screened population increased significantly with age, with a prevalence of 83% (390/468) in those <65 years, and 93% in those ≥65 years (416/449) (Chi-square test, $p=0.0001$). The rate of NP was high in males (90%, 439/486) and females (85%, 367/431), but significantly greater in males (Chi-square test, $p=0.02$). Rates of NP were again high in all ethnic groups (≥80%).

Also in this trial, there was a consistent increase in the proportion of patients with NP in the older age category. However, the prevalence in younger patients was still high, with 66–83% of screened patients with nocturia completing an FVC being affected.

In this study, 89% (141/158) of the patients receiving BPH and/or OAB medication at screening had NP, and 88% (665/759) of those who were not receiving OAB/BPH medication had NP. Although this trial did not exclude patients treated for BPH and OAB, it is possible that screening failures enriched the sample for patients with NP relative to the general nocturia population. However, of the screened population, NP was present in ≥57% of patients, if those without diary data were assumed not to have NP. Therefore, even in the most conservative estimate, the majority of patients with nocturia had NP.

NP is an under-recognized condition and may often be overlooked as a likely cause of nocturia, leading to inaccurate diagnosis and inadequate treatment. The latter was reflected in this trial, wherein around 20% of patients with nocturia were receiving concomitant treatment for OAB and/or BPH. However, nocturia had persisted, leading to their inclusion in the study, and 89% of patients receiving treatment for these conditions had NP. Subsequent exploratory efficacy analyses in the trial [40] found that antidiuretic treatment reduced nocturia equally effectively in patients with and without concomitant OAB and/or BPH medication. The multifactorial nature of nocturia and the value of voiding diaries as simple but effective tools for the identification of patients with NP and/or small voided volumes are therefore highlighted.

Hyponatremia

Desmopressin was well tolerated in all studies and treatment-related adverse event rates were similar to placebo during the double-blind phases. Hyponatremia is the only potentially serious adverse event associated with desmopressin use. Cases are rare and the primary predictor is increasing age. Initiation of desmopressin is therefore currently not indicated for patients aged ≥65 years. The mechanisms behind desmopressin-induced hyponatremia are well understood, and serum sodium monitoring at baseline and early in treatment in older patients can greatly reduce their risk of developing the condition.

Conclusions

Studies with desmopressin showed that NP (defined in accordance with ICS definition) is a major contributing factor to nocturia, with a prevalence between 76% (Noctopus trials) and 88% (USA and Canada Trial) in patients screened for clinical trials who provided evaluable diary data. Additionally, the data indicate that although the prevalence of NP increased with age, it was present in the majority of subjects both under and over 65 years of age (66–83% of <65 years and 90–93% of ≥65 years). The high prevalence of NP found in all trials and all subgroups suggests that this is a leading cause of nocturia in men and women of all ages. Furthermore, since these trials were carried out in Europe and the USA/Canada across several ethnic groups, the relevance of NP for patients across the world is highlighted.

NP is an under-recognized condition and may often be overlooked as a likely cause of nocturia, leading to inaccurate diagnosis and inadequate treatment. The latter was reflected in the USA and Canada Trial, wherein around 20% of patients with nocturia were receiving concomitant treatment for OAB and/or BPH. However, nocturia had persisted, leading to their inclusion in the study, and 89% of patients receiving treatment for these conditions had NP. Subsequent exploratory efficacy analyses in the trial [24] found that antidiuretic treatment reduced nocturia equally effectively in patients with and without concomitant OAB and/or BPH medication. The multifactorial nature of nocturia and the value of voiding diaries as simple but effective tools for the identification of patients with NP and/or small voided volumes are therefore highlighted.

Although the USA and Canada Trial did not exclude patients treated for BPH and OAB, it is possible that screening failures enriched the sample for patients with NP relative to the general nocturia population. However, of the screened population, NP was present in ≥57% of patients, if those without diary data were assumed not to have NP. Therefore, even in the most conservative estimate, the majority of patients with nocturia had NP. Likewise, in the NOCTUPUS trials, ≥64% of subjects had NP, if those without evaluable data were assumed not to have NP. These findings are consistent with previous reports in the literature regarding the high prevalence of NP in patients with nocturia [13–15, 25] and the suboptimal results of treating nocturia with traditional OAB and BPH therapies [26, 27]. It should be noted that if a more conservative definition of nocturnal polyuria is applied to these populations (see Chap. 4), the prevalence of nocturnal polyuria will be seen to be less dramatic than that reported in this chapter.

The potential for inadequate diagnosis in patients with NP is twofold: first, some patients may be inaccurately diagnosed with OAB or BPH because this is the traditional assumption for patients with LUTS; second, some patients may indeed have OAB or BPH, but in combination with NP. The danger for these patients is that NP will go undetected, since clinicians may be more comfortable with the (also accurate) OAB or BPH diagnosis. This, therefore, has a major impact on nocturia therapy, indicating a need to consider this condition – which can have serious consequences for the health and well-being of patients – as a distinct clinical entity, often with a multifactorial pathogenesis, and sometimes independent from other LUTS [41–46]. Following exclusion of other major conditions such as neurogenic disorders, nocturia deserves full evaluation using an FVC to ascertain whether 24-h voiding volumes are excessive (24-h polyuria), or volumes are excessive only at night (NP), or there are small voided volumes (bladder storage problems), or whether a combination of these factors is present. Treatment offered should be directed toward the specific cause(s) identified in each patient to increase the likelihood of achieving clinically meaningful reduction in nocturia.

References

1. Van Kerrebroeck P, Abrams P, Chaikin D, Donovan J, Fonda D, Jackson S, et al. The standardisation of terminology in nocturia: report from the Standardisation Sub-committee of the International Continence Society. Neurourol Urodyn. 2002;21:179.
2. Tikkinen KA, Johnson TM, Tammela TL, Sintonen H, Haukka J, Huhtala H. Nocturia frequency, bother, and quality of life: how often is too often? A population-based study in Finland. Eur Urol. 2010;57:488.
3. Fiske J, Scarpero HM, Xue X, Nitti VW. Degree of bother caused by nocturia in women. Neurourol Urodyn. 2004;23:130.
4. Sagnier PP, MacFarlane G, Teillac P, Botto H, Richard F, Boyle P. Impact of symptoms of prostatism on level of bother and quality of life of men in the French community. J Urol. 1995;153:669.
5. van Dijk MM, Wijkstra H, Debruyne FM, de la Rosette JJ, Michel MC. The role of nocturia in the quality of life of men with lower urinary tract symptoms. BJU Int. 2009;104:143.
6. Bliwise DL, Foley DJ, Vitiello MV, Ansari FP, Ancoli-Israel S, Walsh JK. Nocturia and disturbed sleep in the elderly. Sleep Med. 2008;10:540.
7. Bing MH, Moller LA, Jennum P, Mortensen S, Skovgaard LT, Lose G. Prevalence and bother of nocturia, and causes of sleep interruption in a Danish population of men and women aged 60–80 years. BJU Int. 2006;98:599.
8. Irwin DE, Milsom I, Hunskaar S, Reilly K, Kopp Z, Herschorn S, et al. Population-based survey of urinary incontinence, overactive bladder, and other lower urinary tract symptoms in five countries: results of the EPIC Study. Eur Urol. 2006;50:1306.
9. Bosch JL, Weiss JP. The prevalence and causes of nocturia. J Urol. 2010;184:440.
10. Ancoli-Israel S, Bliwise D, Norgaard J. The effect of nocturia on sleep. Sleep Med Rev. 2010;36:254.
11. Nakagawa H, Niu K, Hozawa A, Ikeda Y, Kaiho Y, Ohmori-Matsuda K, et al. Impact of nocturia on bone fracture and mortality in older individuals: a Japanese longitudinal cohort study. J Urol. 2010;184:1413.
12. Weiss JP, Weinberg AC, Blaivas JG. New aspects of the classification of nocturia. Curr Urol Rep. 2008;9:362.
13. Chang SC, Lin AT, Chen KK, Chang LS. Multifactorial nature of male nocturia. Urology. 2006;67:541.
14. Brubaker L, FitzGerald MP. Nocturnal polyuria and nocturia relief in patients treated with solifenacin for overactive bladder symptoms. Int Urogynecol J Pelvic Floor Dysfunct. 2007;18:737.
15. Koseoglu HO, Aslan G, Ozdemir I, Esen A. Nocturnal polyuria in patients with lower urinary tract symptoms and response to alpha-blocker therapy. Urology. 2006;67:1188.
16. Schneider T, de la Rosette JJ, Michel MC. Nocturia: a non-specific but important symptom of urological disease. Int J Urol. 2009;16:249.

17. Klingler HC, Heidler H, Madersbacher H, Primus G. Nocturia: an Austrian study on the multifactorial etiology of this symptom. Neurourol Urodyn. 2009;28:427.
18. Yoshimura K, Ohara H, Ichioka K, Terada N, Matsui Y, Terai A, et al. Nocturia and benign prostatic hyperplasia. Urology. 2003;61:786.
19. Kujubu DA, Aboseif SR. An overview of nocturia and the syndrome of nocturnal polyuria in the elderly. Nat Clin Pract Nephrol. 2008;4:426.
20. Abrams P, Mattiasson A, Van Kerrebroeck P, Robertson G. Is nocturnal polyuria a key factor in nocturia? Neurourol Urodyn. 2004;23:466.
21. van Kerrebroeck PE, Rezapour M, Cortesse A, Thuroff J, Riis A, Nørgaard JP. Desmopressin in the treatment of nocturia: a double-blind, placebo-controlled study. Eur Urol. 2007;52:221.
22. Andersson K, Chapple C, Cardozo L, Cruz F, Hashim H, Michel M. Pharmacological treatment of urinary incontinence. Report from the fourth international continence on incontinence. Health Publications Ltd; 2009.
23. Rittig S, Jensen AR, Jensen KT, Pedersen EB. Effect of food intake on the pharmacokinetics and antidiuretic activity of oral desmopressin (DDAVP) in hydrated normal subjects. Clin Endocrinol. 1998;48:235.
24. Vande Walle JG, Bogaert GA, Mattsson S, et al. A new fast-melting oral formulation of desmopressin: a pharmacodynamic study in children with primary nocturnal enuresis. BJU Int. 2006;97:603.
25. Richardson DW, Robinson AG. Desmopressin. Ann Intern Med. 1985;103:228.
26. Brink HS, Derkx FH, Boomsma F, et al. Effects of DDAVP on renal hemodynamics and renin secretion in subjects with essential hypertension. Clin Nephrol. 1994;42:95–101.
27. Robertson GL, Norgaard JP. Renal regulation of urine volume: potential implications for nocturia. BJU Int. 2002;90:7–10.
28. Suchowersky O, Furtado S, Rohs G. Beneficial effect of intranasal desmopressin for nocturnal polyuria in Parkinson's disease. Mov Disord. 1995;10:337.
29. Mansson W, Sundin T, Gullberg B. Evaluation of a synthetic vasopressin analogue for treatment of nocturia in benign prostatic hypertrophy. A double-blind study. Scand J Urol Nephrol. 1980;14:139.
30. Hilton P, Hertogs K, Stanton SL. The use of desmopressin (DDAVP) for nocturia in women with multiple sclerosis. J Neurol Neurosurg Psychiatry. 1983;46:854.
31. Kinn AC, Larsson PO. Desmopressin: a new principle for symptomatic treatment of urgency and incontinence in patients with multiple sclerosis. Scand J Urol Nephrol. 1990;24:109.
32. Valiquette G, Herbert J, Maede-D'Alisera P. Desmopressin in the management of nocturia in patients with multiple sclerosis. A double-blind, crossover trial. Arch Neurol. 1996;53:1270.
33. Fredrikson S. Nasal spray desmopressin treatment of bladder dysfunction in patients with multiple sclerosis. Acta Neurol Scand. 1996;94:31.
34. Hilton P, Stanton SL. The use of desmopressin (DDAVP) in nocturnal urinary frequency in the female. Br J Urol. 1982;54:252.
35. Andersson KE, Appell R, Cardozo L, et al. Pharmacological treatment of urinary incontinence. Plymouth, UK: Plymbridge Distributors Ltd.; 2005.
36. Yoong HF, Sundaram MB, Aida Z. Prevalence of nocturnal polyuria in patients with benign prostatic hyperplasia. Med J Malaysia. 2005;60:294.
37. Johnson TM, Burrows PK, Kusek JW, Nyberg LM, Tenover JL, Lepor H, et al. The effect of doxazosin, finasteride and combination therapy on nocturia in men with benign prostatic hyperplasia. J Urol. 2007;178:2045.
38. Rackley R, Weiss JP, Rovner ES, Wang JT, Guan Z. Nighttime dosing with tolterodine reduces overactive bladder-related nocturnal micturitions in patients with overactive bladder and nocturia. Urology. 2006;67:731.
39. Weiss JP, Snyder J, Ellison W, Belkoff L. Klein. Fast-dissolving desmopressin (Melt) is well tolerated in nocturia: results of a randomized, placebo-controlled study. J Urol. 2010;183:e589.
40. Weiss J, Zinner N, Daneshgari F, Klein B, Norgaard J, Ancoli-Israel S. Desmopressin orally disintegrating tablet effectively reduces symptoms of nocturia and prolongs undisturbed sleep

in patients with nocturia: results of a randomized placebo-controlled study. International Continence Society; 2010, abstract 198.
41. Yu HJ, Chen FY, Huang PC, Chen TH, Chie WC, Liu CY. Impact of nocturia on symptom-specific quality of life among community-dwelling adults aged 40 years and older. Urology. 2006;67:713.
42. Hernandez FC, Ristol PJ, Estivill E, Batista Miranda JE, Lopez Aramburu MA. Importance of nocturia and its impact on quality of sleep and quality of life in patient with benign prostatic hyperplasia. Actas Urol Esp. 2007;31:262.
43. Asplund R. Nocturia: consequences for sleep and daytime activities and associated risks. Eur Urol Suppl. 2005;3:24.
44. Mattiasson A, Abrams P, Van Kerrebroeck P, Walter S, Weiss J. Efficacy of desmopressin in the treatment of nocturia: a double-blind placebo-controlled study in men. BJU Int. 2002;89:855.
45. Lose G, Lalos O, Freeman RM, van Kerrebroeck P. Efficacy of desmopressin (Minirin) in the treatment of nocturia: a double-blind placebo-controlled study in women. Am J Obstet Gynecol. 2003;189:1106.
46. Lose G, Mattiasson A, Walter S, et al. Clinical experiences with desmopressin for long-term treatment of nocturia. J Urol. 2004;172:1021.

Chapter 10
Nocturia in the Elderly

Catherine E. DuBeau and Johnson F. Tsui

Keywords Nocturia • Elderly • Lower urinary tract symptoms (LUTS) • Nocturia Nocturnal Enuresis and Sleep-interruption Questionnaire (NNES-Q) • Quality of life • Healthcare costs • Morbidity • Comorbid disease • Falls • Mortality

Introduction

Nocturia is a part of life for most older persons, especially men, nearly 90% of whom experience at least one episode of nighttime voiding [1]. It is often cited as one of the most bothersome of lower urinary tract symptoms (LUTS) [2, 3]. Unlike the other common LUTS, nocturia can cause significant morbidity and even mortality for elderly persons.

At the same time, our understanding of nocturia in older persons is complicated by how this condition has been defined. The ICS definition of nocturia, the number of voids recorded during a night's sleep with each void preceded and followed by sleep [4], assumes that "a night's sleep" is relatively stable and consistently understood by patients. However, older persons spend more time in bed before falling asleep [5, 6], and may count time in bed rather than time asleep when self-reporting nocturia. Older persons also experience more awakenings from sleep independent of comorbidity [7, 8]. When these awakenings are combined with age-associated shifts in diurnal urine output to later in the day and night, nocturia becomes essentially normal. In older persons, the number of nocturia episodes also should be

C.E. DuBeau, MD (✉)
Division of Geriatric Medicine, University of Massachusetts Medical Center, Worcester, MA, USA
e-mail: Catherine.Dubeau@umassmemorial.org

J.F. Tsui, BS
SUNY Downstate College of Medicine, Brooklyn, NY, USA

placed in context of actual hours asleep and/or in bed, which can vary greatly. For example, three episodes of nocturia over 6 h likely have a different pathophysiology and impact than three episodes over 12 h.

Causes of Nocturia in Elderly Men and Women

Analogous to the situation with urinary incontinence in older persons, the etiology of nocturia is similar for younger persons and healthier elderly. However, among older, less healthy, and vulnerable elderly, the etiology of nocturia is best conceptualized by a syndromic and not a disease model of illness, in which nocturia is a multifactorial condition that is caused by the accumulation of impairments in multiple systems, the interactions between them, and increased vulnerability for minor perturbations to cause problematic symptoms [9, 10]. For example, when an older man with diabetes mellitus, mild venous stasis, and pre-existing age-related nocturnal polyuria is prescribed prednisone for treatment of a COPD exacerbation, bothersome nocturia of several episodes per night can result from worsening peripheral edema and hyperglycemia caused by the steroid.

The major factors underlying nocturia in older persons are altered and/or disturbed sleep, nocturnal polyuria, and an increased prevalence of lower urinary disorders causing relatively low bladder capacity (Table 10.1) [10, 11]. A number of conditions and medications may affect several of these domains, leading to an additive impact on nocturia. For example, congestive heart failure and steroids can cause both disturbed sleep and nocturnal polyuria.

Quality-of-Life Impact

Nocturia is one of the most bothersome of symptoms related to BPH in men and OAB in women [2, 12]. Patients characterize it as unpredictable, "debilitating, frustrating, distressing, and puzzling," and leading to poor self-image ("feel old"), worry about nighttime falls, and poor self-rated health [13–15].

The standard instrument for assessment of the impact of nocturia is the ICIQ-NQOL. The questionnaire includes 13 questions on specific impact, bother, and quality-of-life effect from nocturia, with two subscales, bother/concern, and sleep/energy [16]. ICIQ-NQOL was derived and validated only in men, although a focus group study suggests it has content validity among women [14]. Also, ICI-NQOL does not address key content areas for older persons (feeling older and fear of falling)

Unlike the ICIQ-NQOL, the Nocturia Nocturnal Enuresis and Sleep-interruption Questionnaire (NNES-Q) was validated in older men and women (aged 60–80 years) [17]. It is not strictly a QoL or bother instrument, as other than frequency of nocturia and related bother, it captures patients' perceptions of the

Table 10.1 Common causes of nocturia in older persons

Altered and/or disturbed sleep
  Age-related changes in circadian rhythms, REM sleep, and sleep duration
  Sleep apnea
  Bed partner (including roommate in long-term care)
  Medications [43]
    Steroids
    Cardiovascular drugs: statins, beta-blockers, ACE inhibitors, amiodarone
    Psychoactive drugs: serotonin re-uptake inhibitors, antipsychotics
    Phenytoin
    Anti-Parkinsonian agents
    Leukotriene receptor antagonists
    Caffeine
    Alcohol
  Depression
  Alzheimer's disease
  Movement disorders: Parkinson's, restless leg syndrome
  Congestive heart failure
  Pain

Nocturnal polyuria
  Age-related
  Sleep apnea
  Uncontrolled diabetes mellitus
  Uncontrolled hypertension
  Hypertensive kidney disease
  Peripheral edema
    Venous stasis
    Congestive heart failure
    Medications: pyridine calcium channel blockers, steroids, NSAIDs, thiazolidinediones, GABA-nergic agents

Lower urinary disorders associated with low functional bladder capacity
  Detrusor overactivity
  Bladder outlet obstruction
  Chronic: Interstitial, radiation, bacterial
  Neurogenic bladder/urethra

cause of nocturnal awakening, and the presence of incontinence and falls. Using this instrument, Bing et al. found: a significant association between QoL and the frequency and bother of nocturia episodes; a greater impact in the younger elderly; and greater bother among women compared to men. Such a gender difference has not been consistently found in other studies, although some included younger patients [17].

There appears to be a threshold effect at three episodes per night for nocturia-associated bother and quality-of-life impairment. In a population-based study, bother was reported by patients with at least two episodes, and moderate to severe bother among those with a least three episodes [18]. Similar threshold for significant bother of at least three episodes has been reported for older women with LUTS as well [19].

Family and Caregiver Burden

Regardless of age, bed partners of persons with nocturia are subject to awakenings and sleep deprivation, leading to sleeping in separate beds, which carries a powerful symbolic significance. Among the frail elderly, the impact of nocturia on caregivers can be particularly acute. Sleep deprivation may result less from sleep interruption than the need to stay awake for continual monitoring, especially when there is a risk of falls: "I was just like a mother with a sick child. Your ear is cocked and you have a very shallow sleep, just sort of in and out of sleep like this the whole time, with no deep sleep at all. Well, I got so run down that I was nearly falling down." [20] Caregivers of patients with dementia and nocturia have significantly higher rates of depression and chronic illness [21].

Healthcare Costs

Few studies have specifically addressed the economic impact of nocturia separate from other LUTS and urinary incontinence. One population-based study found that persons with at least three episodes of nocturia had higher total medical costs (OR 1.26, $p=0.0002$), reflecting a combination of greater number of hospitalization days (OR 1.53, $p<0.001$), and higher outpatient and inpatient medical costs (respectively, OR 1.13, $p=0.024$, and OR 1.45, $p=0.003$) [22]. It is striking that there is a similar threshold effect at ≥3 episodes for QoL, bother, and economic impact.

Sleep Disturbance

By definition, persons with nocturia experience sleep interruption, which can then lead to insomnia and poor sleep quality. Nocturia is a major risk factor for self-reported insomnia and poor sleep, following depression, stroke, and arthritis [23]. In a population-based telephone survey among older persons, nocturia was listed as a self-perceived cause of interrupted sleep "every night or almost every night" by 53%, and was an independent predictor of self-reported insomnia and reduced sleep quality [24]. Poor sleep quality and daytime sleepiness are especially marked when nocturia is followed by difficulty going back to sleep.

For example, in a population-based study of older persons, Asplund found significant correlations between having ≥3 nocturnal voids and poor sleep (OR, 2.6, CI, 2.1–3.2), sequelae after stroke (OR, 2.0, CI, 1.1–3.6), irregular heartbeats (OR, 1.6, CI, 1.2–2.1) and diabetes (OR, 1.5, CI, 1.1–2.3) [25]. Another population-based survey demonstrated a significant relationship in men between any nocturia and bladder/prostate cancer, BPH, hypertension, cerebrovascular disease, diabetes, treatment for LUTS, and moderate alcohol consumption [26].

Morbidity

Comorbid Disease. Nocturia in older persons is associated with a range of comorbid conditions, and causal relationships between them may be bidirectional. For example, nocturia is associated with worsening hypertension and impaired nocturnal blood pressure control [27, 28], possibly a result of the observed increased nighttime plasma catecholamine levels and increased daytime and nighttime plasma natriuretic peptide levels [29]. At the same time, worsening hypertension is associated with congestive heart failure, which leads to nocturnal polyuria and nocturia, and this cycle may continue. The association between nocturia and cardiovascular disease may be mediated by obesity; in women, nocturnal eating and BMI increase in parallel with the number of nocturia episodes [30]. Men with depressive symptoms have nearly three times higher risk of having moderate to severe nocturia compared with men without such symptoms, but the directionality is unclear [31]. Sleep deprivation may be an important covariate mediating the association in several directions: depression-associated sleep interruption and awakening may lead to nocturnal bathroom trips, whereas nocturia-related sleep interruption may cause or worsen depressive symptoms.

Obstructive sleep apnea (OSA) is increasingly appreciated as an important cause of nocturnal polyuria and resulting nocturia. Moreover, treatment of sleep apnea with nasal CPAP reduces nocturia and improves quality of life, in both younger and older patients. In older men with OSA, the presence of nocturia is associated with higher BMI, worse apnea and hypoxia, and worse health-related QoL [32]. Diagnostic clues to the presence of sleep apnea include obesity, poorly controlled hypertension, nocturnal polyuria, morning headache, and, importantly, history from a bed partner. Detection and treatment of sleep apnea will result in not only decreased nocturia but also decreased cardiovascular and all-cause mortality.

Other conditions and factors associated with nocturia appear to have specific causal relationships. For example, moderate alcohol consumption and poorly controlled diabetes can lead to nocturnal polyuria [33]. Pain, restless leg syndrome, Alzheimer's disease, and Parkinson's disease can lead to increased awakenings and subsequent trips to the bathroom. In patients with pain, and in diabetics with poor glycemic control, the causality is less clear.

Falls. Among the elderly, falls are perhaps the most feared complication of nocturia. Most nighttime falls are associated with trips to the bathroom, versus only 20% of daytime falls [34]. Nocturia is associated with a 25% increase in the risk of a fall, with a parallel increase between number of nocturia episodes and falls [34]. Poor lighting and visibility, slippery hard bathroom surfaces, and nocturia-associated incontinence combine to make nocturia-related falls result in both fractures and head injury. In older men, those with at least two episodes of nocturia had three times the risk of hip fracture compared to men without nocturia. Among men with nocturia, the risk of facture increased with the number of nocturia episodes [35].

Mortality

Of special concern is the association between nocturia and mortality in older persons. In a population-based study, older men with at least three episodes of nocturia had a death rate 1.9 (CI 1.4, 2.6) times more than the whole group, with an increase of 3.4% vs. 1.9% per 6 months ($P<0.001$) [36]. In the multivariate analysis, nocturia of at least three episodes was independently associated with death. Similar associations were not observed among older women. The increased mortality associated with nocturia may be mediated by poor sleep efficiency, independent of comorbidity; [24] comorbid conditions (e.g., cardiovascular disease and sleep apnea); and other sequelae such as hip fracture.

Issues in Nocturia Treatment in Older Adults

Despite increased elucidation of the multifactorial, syndromic basis of nocturia in older persons, in clinical practice nocturia is commonly assumed to be due to BPH in men and OAB in women. These assumptions can lead to missed opportunities to diagnose significantly morbid diseases (e.g., sleep apnea). Misdirected therapy with alpha-blockers, 5-alpha reductase inhibitors, and bladder antimuscarinics not only fails to improve nocturia but can also contribute to polypharmacy, adverse drug effects (ADEs), and drug–drug interactions, with subsequent impact on medication compliance, morbidity, and hospitalizations [37–40].

Inappropriate use of medications in older persons can lead to a phenomenon called the "prescribing cascade," [37, 41] in which a medication is used to treat what is actually an ADE from another medication. A pertinent example with nocturia is inappropriate use of antimuscarinics for presumed OAB/DO in an older man, which can cause an increase in PVR leading to a decrease in functional bladder capacity, worsening nocturia, and subsequent addition of an alpha-blocker. In such a case, the alpha-blocker is essentially being used to treat an ADE, leading to persistent bothersome symptoms and additional polypharmacy.

The evaluation of nocturia in older persons should include review of existing comorbid conditions and medications, and a history and physical examination that specifically looks for common causes of sleep disturbance and nocturnal polyuria (Table 10.1) [10].

Unfortunately, there is little level 1 evidence for successful treatment of nocturia in older persons (Table 10.2). Antimuscarinic trials have either not included large numbers of older adults or shown only very small net benefit over placebo (absolute difference of 0–0.3 episodes/night) [42]. There is robust randomized controlled trial evidence that DDAVP causes significant hyponatremia in the elderly, and should *not* be used. Otherwise, there are only some clinical "pearls" supported by less robust trials and/or expert opinion for judicious use of timed diuretics, antimuscarinics, or low-dose, short-acting sedative hypnotics, depending upon the likely underlying etiology of nocturia.

Table 10.2 Evidence-based recommendations for the treatment of nocturia in older persons [10]

- Late afternoon administration of a diuretic may reduce nocturia in persons with lower extremity venous insufficiency or congestive heart failure unresponsive to other interventions (Level 2)
- If OAB, detrusor overactivity, and/or urgency incontinence is felt to be a major contributor to nocturia, antimuscarinic agents should be considered (Level 3)
- If nocturia is due to insomnia alone, then a very short acting sedative hypnotic may be considered (Level 3)
- DDAVP should not be used in frail elderly because of the risk of hyponatremia (Level 1)

Summary

Nocturia is a highly prevalent symptom in older persons, the pathophysiology of which is multifactorial and syndromic. It causes significant impact on the quality of life of affected patients as well as their caregivers, and is associated with high comorbidity and even death. Failure to consider the many common causes of disturbed sleep and nocturnal polyuria in this age group will lead to not only inappropriate treatment and persistent nocturia but also polypharmacy and missed opportunities to detect significant underlying conditions. Treatment of nocturia initially targets contributing comorbidity, conditions, and medications. Treatment of nocturia due to detrusor overactivity with antimuscarinics has limited efficacy, and DDAVP should be used judiciously or avoided in this age group.

References

1. Malmsten UG, Milsom I, Molander U, et al. Urinary incontinence and lower urinary tract symptoms: an epidemiological study of men aged 45 to 99 years. J Urol. 1997;158:1733.
2. DuBeau CE, Yalla SV, Resnick NM. Implications of the most bothersome prostatism symptom for clinical care and outcomes research. J Am Geriatr Soc. 1995;43:985.
3. Eckhardt MD, van Venrooij GE, van Melick HH, et al. Prevalence and bothersomeness of lower urinary tract symptoms in benign prostatic hyperplasia and their impact on well-being. J Urol. 2001;166:563.
4. Van Kerrebroeck P, Abrams P, Chaikin D, et al. The standardization of terminology in nocturia: report from the Standardization Subcommittee of the International Continence Society. BJU Int. 2002;90 Suppl 3:11.
5. Bliwise DL. Sleep in normal aging and dementia. Sleep. 1993;16:40.
6. Ohayon MM, Zulley J, Guilleminault C, et al. How age and daytime activities are related to insomnia in the general population: consequences for older people. J Am Geriatr Soc. 2001;49:360.
7. Webb WB. Sleep in older persons: sleep structures of 50- to 60-year-old men and women. J Gerontol. 1982;37:581.
8. Dijk DJ, Duffy JF, Czeisler CA. Age-related increase in awakenings: impaired consolidation of nonREM sleep at all circadian phases. Sleep. 2001;24:565.
9. Inouye SK, Studenski S, Tinetti ME, et al. Geriatric syndromes: clinical, research, and policy implications of a core geriatric concept. J Am Geriatr Soc. 2007;55:780.
10. DuBeau CE, Kuchel GA, Johnson 2nd T, et al. Incontinence in the frail elderly: report from the 4th International Consultation on Incontinence. Neurourol Urodyn. 2010;29:165.

11. Weiss JP, Blaivas JG. Nocturia. J Urol. 2000;163:5.
12. Coyne KS, Zhou Z, Bhattacharyya SK, et al. The prevalence of nocturia and its effect on health-related quality of life and sleep in a community sample in the USA. BJU Int. 2003;92:948.
13. Newman AB, Spiekerman CF, Enright P, et al. Daytime sleepiness predicts mortality and cardiovascular disease in older adults. The Cardiovascular Health Study Research Group. J Am Geriatr Soc. 2000;48:115.
14. Mock LL, Parmelee PA, Kutner N, et al. Content validation of symptom-specific nocturia quality-of-life instrument developed in men: issues expressed by women, as well as men. Urology. 2008;72:736.
15. Booth JM, Lawrence M, O'Neill K, et al. Exploring older peoples' experiences of nocturia: a poorly recognised urinary condition that limits participation. Disabil Rehabil. 2010;32:765.
16. Abraham L, Hareendran A, Mills IW, et al. Development and validation of a quality-of-life measure for men with nocturia. Urology. 2004;63:481.
17. Bing MH, Moller LA, Jennum P, et al. Validity and reliability of a questionnaire for evaluating nocturia, nocturnal enuresis and sleep-interruptions in an elderly population. Eur Urol. 2006;49:710.
18. Tikkinen KA, Johnson 2nd TM, Tammela TL, et al. Nocturia frequency, bother, and quality of life: how often is too often? A population-based study in Finland. Eur Urol. 2010;57:488.
19. Lowenstein L, Brubaker L, Kenton K, et al. Prevalence and impact of nocturia in a urogynecologic population. Int Urogynecol J Pelvic Floor Dysfunct. 2007;18:1049.
20. Cassells C, Watt E. The impact of incontinence on older spousal caregivers. J Adv Nurs. 2003;42:607.
21. Canadian Study of Health and Aging Working Group. Patterns and health effects of caring for people with dementia: the impact of changing cognitive and residential status. Gerontologist. 2002;42:643.
22. Nakagawa H, Ikeda Y, Kaiho Y, et al. Impact of nocturia on medical care use and its costs in an elderly population: 30 month prospective observation of National Health Insurance Beneficiaries in Japan. Neurourol Urodyn. 2009;28:930.
23. Dew MA, Hoch CC, Buysse DJ, et al. Healthy older adults' sleep predicts all-cause mortality at 4 to 19 years of follow-up. Psychosom Med. 2003;65:63.
24. Bliwise DL, Foley DJ, Vitiello MV, et al. Nocturia and disturbed sleep in the elderly. Sleep Med. 2009;10:540.
25. Asplund R. Nocturia in relation to sleep, somatic diseases and medical treatment in the elderly. BJU Int. 2002;90:533.
26. Gourova LW, van de Beek C, Spigt MG, et al. Predictive factors for nocturia in elderly men: a cross-sectional study in 21 general practices. BJU Int. 2006;97:528.
27. Agarwal R, Light RP, Bills JE, et al. Nocturia, nocturnal activity, and nondipping. Hypertension. 2009;54:646.
28. Asplund R. Diuresis pattern, plasma vasopressin and blood pressure in healthy elderly persons with nocturia and nocturnal polyuria. Neth J Med. 2002;60:276.
29. Sugaya K, Nishijima S, Oda M, et al. Biochemical and body composition analysis of nocturia in the elderly. Neurourol Urodyn. 2008;27:205.
30. Asplund R. Obesity in elderly people with nocturia: cause or consequence? Can J Urol. 2007;14:3424.
31. Hakkinen JT, Shiri R, Koskimaki J, et al. Depressive symptoms increase the incidence of nocturia: Tampere Aging Male Urologic Study (TAMUS). J Urol. 2008;179:1897.
32. Guilleminault C, Lin CM, Goncalves MA, et al. A prospective study of nocturia and the quality of life of elderly patients with obstructive sleep apnea or sleep onset insomnia. J Psychosom Res. 2004;56:511.
33. Tikkinen KA, Auvinen A, Johnson 2nd TM, et al. A systematic evaluation of factors associated with nocturia – the population-based FINNO study. Am J Epidemiol. 2009;170:361.
34. Endeshaw Y. Correlates of self-reported nocturia among community-dwelling older adults. J Gerontol A Biol Sci Med Sci. 2009;64:142.

35. Temml C, Ponholzer A, Gutjahr G, et al. Nocturia is an age-independent risk factor for hip-fractures in men. Neurourol Urodyn. 2009;28:949.
36. Asplund R. Mortality in the elderly in relation to nocturnal micturition. BJU Int. 1999;84:297.
37. Gurwitz JH, Avorn J. The ambiguous relation between aging and adverse drug reactions. Ann Intern Med. 1991;114:956.
38. Kaufman DW, Kelly JP, Rosenberg L, et al. Recent patterns of medication use in the ambulatory adult population of the United States: the Slone survey. JAMA. 2002;287:337.
39. Schmader K, Hanlon JT, Weinberger M, et al. Appropriateness of medication prescribing in ambulatory elderly patients. J Am Geriatr Soc. 1994;42:1241.
40. Lipton HL, Bero LA, Bird JA, et al. The impact of clinical pharmacists' consultations on physicians' geriatric drug prescribing. A randomized controlled trial. Med Care. 1992;30:646.
41. Avorn J, Gurwitz JH, Rochon P. Principles of pharmacology. In: Cassel CK, Leipzip RM, Cohen HJ, et al., editors. Geriatric medicine: an evidence-based approach. 4th ed. New York: Springer; 2003. p. 65–81.
42. Johnson TM, Burridge A, Issa MM, et al. The relationship between the action of arginine vasopressin and responsiveness to oral desmopressin in older men: a pilot study. J Am Geriatr Soc. 2007;55:562.
43. Harbison J. Sleep disorders in older people. Age Ageing. 2002;31:6.

Chapter 11
Nocturia: Treatment with Alternative Therapies

Duong D. Tu and Franklin C. Lowe

Keywords Alternative therapies • Nocturia • Lifestyle changes • Supplements • Plant extracts • Permixon • Finasteride • Tamsulosin

In a time of overeagerness toward the use of prescription medications to treat diseases and symptoms, of which benign prostatic hyperplasia (BPH) and nocturia are not exempt, it is easy to disregard or minimize the importance that lifestyle changes can play in overall management. Indeed, for patients who have mild symptoms that are not particularly bothersome, such behavioral modification may be preferable in view of its general safety and the perception of cost-effectiveness.

Lifestyle Changes

The first of these lifestyle changes are behavioral modifications targeted at the alleviation of factors that may exacerbate BPH symptoms. The simplest modification is fluid restriction. This seemingly intuitive change can have a significant impact on nocturia, and patients often do not realize the extent of their intake, especially post-dinner/pre-bedtime, until they are specifically asked during a careful history. The intake of diuretics, such as caffeinated beverages and alcohol, can, in some patients, be quite substantial and the quantity, as well as timing of consumption of such beverages, should be assessed. These effects sometimes are already recognized by the patients and have changed their "habits" accordingly before presenting to the

D.D. Tu, MD (✉) • F. C. Lowe, MD, MPH
Departments of Urology, Columbia University,
College of Physicians & Surgeons and St Luke's/Roosevelt Hospital Center,
Boston Children's Hospital, New York, NY, USA
e-mail: tu.duong.d@gmail.com

physician's office. However, verification of these habits should be done by the treating physician upon the initial encounter.

Comorbid conditions play a role in nocturia as well. The polyuria associated with poorly controlled diabetes mellitus contribute greatly to nocturnal symptoms, and, moreover, can lead to persistent symptoms, even when causes from BPH have been treated. Patients who take diuretics for hypertension or congestive heart failure also suffer from polyuria, and the simple act of changing the timing of these medications (i.e., from bedtime to morning dosing) can sometimes alleviate nocturia. Of course, these changes should be performed with the primary doctor caring for these illnesses being aware. Indirectly related to these diseases is the issue of lower extremity edema, which develops throughout the day, but with mobilization of that fluid with recumbency at night it becomes another cause of nocturia. This phenomenon can also occur with healthy individuals in the absence of heart disease. Elevation of the feet well before bedtime for fluid mobilization helps to limit the amount of nocturia by increasing the amount of fluid voided prior to bedtime.

Supplements

Inundated by the marketing for the use of supplements, many men begin taking herbal/dietary supplements to alleviate nocturia without the use of "medications." Lured in by perceptions of supplements being "natural," not manufactured in a cold, lifeless lab, relatively "inexpensive," presumptively "safe," and obtainable without a doctor's prescription or office visit, 30–90% of men have used supplements prior to seeking medical treatment in the United States [1, 2]. Patients have easy access to obtaining these supplements lining drug store shelves, and the Internet has made purchasing them and having them delivered to their home even easier.

A variety of herbal supplements are available for the promotion of "prostate health" (Table 11.1).

Table 11.1 Origin of plant extracts/supplements

Common name	Species name
Saw palmetto berry	*Serenoa repens*
African plum tree	*Pygeum africanum*
South African star grass	*Hypoxis rooperi*
Stinging nettle	*Urtica dioica*
Rye pollen	*Secale cereal*
Pumpkin seed	*Cucurbita pepo*
Cactus flower	*Opuntia*
Pine flower	*Pinus*
Spruce	*Picea*

Table 11.2 Proposed mechanisms of action of Saw palmetto berry (SPB)

Anti-androgenic: 5 alpha-reductase inhibition, dihydrotestosterone binding inhibition
Anti-estrogenic: estrogen receptor inhibition
Anti-inflammatory: cyclooxygenase and lipoxygenase enzymatic inhibition
Apoptosis promotion
Anti-proliferative/growth factor inhibition

Mechanisms of Action

The actual "active" substances in these plants are extracts from various components of the plant from the root (South African Star Grass) to the bark (African plum) to the fruit (Saw palmetto berry). Mechanisms of action of these agents have been undergoing intense investigation. There has been an overabundance of in vitro experimental studies using tissue cultures; however, extrapolation of these results to "normal" use is problematic given the supraphysiologic dose used in these studies.

The most widely studied of all of the plant extracts used by patients for nocturia is *Serenoa repens* or Saw palmetto berry (SPB). The exact mechanism of action is unclear, although many suggestions have been made including anti-androgenic, anti-inflammatory, and anti-proliferative action (Table 11.2) [3].

The lipido-sterolic component of *Serenoa repens*, brand named Permixon® (Pierre Fabre Medicament, Castres, France), has been the most intensely studied, and its efficacy will be discussed later in the chapter.

As for the other phytotherapeutic agents, their mechanisms of action are unknown. *Pygeum africanum* (African plum) has demonstrated similar anti-proliferative and anti-inflammatory effects as SPB with an additional protective effect on the obstructed bladder [4, 5]. The other extracts have been less intensely studied but the active components, often the sterol component, are postulated to have similar effects.

Difficulties in Evaluation

Determining the "active" constituent in any of the numerous formulations of phytoextracts is no simple matter. Many of the manufactured products available are combination products with more than one specific plant extract, often touting these "new" combinations as "enhanced" or more effective than their competitors. These extracts are composites of several different chemical molecules including phytosterols, oils, phytoestrogens, and other such compounds. Phytotherapeutics do not undergo as strict regulation by the Food and Drug Administration (FDA) as the pharmaceutical companies for drugs. Indeed, they are regarded as dietary supplements or as a category of foods, and, as such, do not require FDA approval prior to entering the market. The Dietary Supplement Health and Education Act of 1994 (DSHEA) was the result of efforts of the manufacturers of these supplements to restrict the FDA's authority over them. In return, these manufacturers cannot make any claims of their products treating or preventing diseases, although claims that a product influences the structure or function of the body are acceptable. Also, it is a quality requirement that "the dietary supplement consistently meets the established specifications for identity, purity, strength, and composition and has been manufactured, packaged, labeled, and held under conditions to prevent adulteration under section 402(a)(1), (a)(2), (a)(3), and (a)(4) of the Federal Food, Drug, and Cosmetic Act." As discussed below, this is often not the case, and problems with enforcement of such dictates persist.

Product Variability

Since all of these supplements require extraction of the "active" substances from plants which inherently have natural variability, the products on the market are equally as variable. Moreover, there is no standardized method for extraction of these very complex extracts, and, therefore, the extraction process also varies not only between different manufacturers but even within the same manufacturing group. For example, the dosage of saw palmetto berry extract varied from −97% to +140% of the dose stated on the bottle label with half the products having less than 20% of stated dose [6]. One study comparing 14 brands of SPB extract revealed significant variation of the amount of what is considered the "active" elements of the extract, responsible for its purported biologic effects on the prostate [7]. This tremendous variability makes any meaningful comparison between products virtually impossible.

Efficacy

Two published meta-analyses revealed that SPB extract was superior to placebo in improving symptoms of nocturia in patients. One meta-analysis included all placebo-controlled trials; the other examined all the trials involving the lipido-sterolic extract of SPB, Permixon®, specifically [8, 9]. In the more recent latter meta-analysis, it was suggested that Permixon® increases Q_{max} by 1.0 ($P=0.042$) mL/s and reduces the mean number of episodes of nocturia by 0.37 ($P<0.001$) episodes when compared to placebo. There was heterogeneity among the studies, however, and the effect on nocturia in the newer and longer studies was smaller [9].

Recent evidence including a double-blind placebo-controlled randomized trial showed no significant benefit over placebo regarding parameters of the International Prostate Symptom Score (IPSS[1]), peak urinary flow rate, and the Rosen International Index of Erectile Function (IIEF) questionnaire [10]. Newer evidence with similar conclusions, as well as a complete review from the Cochrane Database, will be discussed in a subsequent section of this chapter [11, 12].

---

[1] IPSS/AUASI: validated seven questions on urgency, daytime and nighttime urinary frequency, hesitancy, intermittency, sensation of incomplete voiding, and force of urine stream.

A systematic review and quantitative meta-analysis of the therapeutic efficacy and tolerability of *P. africanum* (African plum) revealed modest but significant overall improvement of nocturia (19%), postvoid residual (24%), and peak urine flow (23%), despite the short duration of the studies and variable study designs. The phytotherapeutic preparations in these studies were not standardized [13]. Larger placebo-controlled trials with longer follow-up, standardized preparations of the extract, and the use of standardized validated measures of efficacy (e.g., AUASI/IPSS) would be needed to adequately demonstrate a true beneficial effect on lower urinary tract symptoms (LUTS) and nocturia.

Permixon, Finasteride, and Tamsulosin

The lipido-sterolic extract of *Serenoa repens* (LSESr), Permixon®, was shown to have an equivalent efficacy to finasteride in patients with benign prostatic hyperplasia (BPH). In a 6-month, double-blind randomized trial, Permixon® at 320 mg daily (160 mg BID) was compared to daily 5 mg of finasteride in 1,098 men with moderate BPH as measured using the International Prostate Symptom Score (IPSS). Changes in the IPSS were used as the primary endpoint in this equivalence study. In addition, peak urinary flow rates and quality of life and sexual function questionnaires were completed at 6, 13, and 26 weeks. In the latter two visits, transrectal/abdominal ultrasound was used to determine prostatic volume and postvoid residual urine. *Both treatment arms had similar decreases in IPSS (−37% Permixon® vs. −39% finasteride), improved quality of life (38 and 41%), and increased peak urinary flow rates (+25 and 30%).* As expected, finasteride decreased prostate volume and serum PSA levels, whereas Permixon® had no significant effect. However, Permixon® was noted to be superior with regard to results of the sexual function questionnaire with fewer complaints of decreased libido and erectile dysfunction [14]. There was no placebo arm in this trial.

Two recent studies have examined the clinical efficacy of Permixon® versus the most commonly used α-blocker, tamsulosin, in the treatment of lower urinary tract symptoms (LUTS) attributable to BPH. The PERMAL study consisted of 704 patients randomized in a 12-month, double-blind trial into two treatment arms: Permixon® 320 mg daily and tamsulosin 0.4 mg daily. *The study demonstrated clinical equivalence between the two groups with respect to decreases in IPSS and LUTS. Likewise, the increase in peak urinary flow rates was not different between the groups. Ejaculation disorders (retrograde or diminished ejaculation) were more frequent in the tamsulosin arm than the Permixon® arm (4.2 vs. 0.6%, respectively; p=0.001).* Otherwise, overall tolerability of the two treatments was similar [15]. A subset analysis was performed for patients with severe LUTS (IPSS>19). At 12 months, IPSS decreased by two more points with Permixon® versus tamsulosin (7.8 vs. 5.8, $p=0.051$) with a greater improvement in irritative symptoms (−2.9 vs. −1.9, $p=0.049$) [16].

A prospective study was designed comparing Permixon® (320 mg daily), tamsulosin (0.4 mg daily), and combined therapy of Permixon® plus tamsulosin in an open-label 6-month study. Twenty patients were included in each treatment arm. *There was no statistical difference in peak urinary flow rates and IPSS between the Permixon® and tamsulosin groups; moreover, there was no additional benefit when they were used in combination.* No adverse effects were observed with Permixon® [17]. This study was limited by its small sample size and short follow-up (6 months).

The lack of a placebo arm renders a determination of individual efficacy for each drug difficult with possible biases of missing data, noncompliance, dropouts, or violation of entry criteria. Therefore, these studies can only state what they ultimately set out to do: prove equivalence between two drugs in the patient populations studied.

Saw Palmetto for Treatment of Enlarged Prostates Trial

The longest placebo-controlled randomized trial to date examined the efficacy of SPB versus placebo over a 12-month period. Two hundred and twenty-five men with moderate-to-severe symptoms of BPH were randomized to a group who received 160 mg twice daily, saw palmetto capsules, or a group who received placebo in similar-appearing gelatin capsules. Given the difficulties as discussed previously with inconsistencies with proportions of content for these extracts, the extract used in this trial was manufactured in one batch, and the proportions of the theoretically "active" substances within the extract were similar to that found in the majority of currently available products as determined by a reference laboratory. Ninety-six percent of the randomized patients completed the study and 91.6% of all study medication was consumed. There was no difference in compliance between the two groups. The study showed no significant difference in American Urological Association Symptom Index (AUASI) scores, BPH Impact Index, maximal urinary flow rate, postvoid residual, or quality of life. Moreover, serum PSA, creatinine, and testosterone levels were similar. *These findings were all consistent in showing no evidence of an effect* [11].

The Cochrane Database of Systematic Reviews published a review "aimed to assess the effects of *Serenoa repens* in the treatment of LUTS consistent with BPH." Trials in the database had to meet criteria for eligibility: randomization of men with symptomatic BPH to *Serenoa repens* in comparison with placebo or other interventions, follow-up of at least 4 weeks, and inclusion of clinical outcomes measured objectively as with urologic symptom scales (AUASI/IPSS) and urodynamic measurements (peak urinary flow rates). *There were no significant differences in improvement of IPSS, nocturia, peak urinary flow, and prostate size* [12].

In conclusion, the highest quality study to date [11] and a systematic review performed by the Cochrane Collaboration group determine that there is no substantive benefit of SPB/*Serenoa repens* versus placebo.

Monitoring Side Effects

As part of the Saw palmetto for treatment of enlarged prostates (STEP) trial, data were collected on adverse events, sexual functioning, and laboratory blood and urine tests. The probability of suffering at least one serious adverse event was not statistically significant to find a difference between the two groups (SPB vs. placebo). Also, none of these serious events, including cardiovascular incidents, elective orthopedic procedures, or serious gastrointestinal problems, were assessed as related to the study medicine. *Similarly, assessment of the likelihood for experiencing at least one "nonserious" adverse event was also not significantly different between the two groups.* The nonserious adverse events were categorized by organ systems and the most commonly reported ones were musculoskeletal (e.g., joint pain and myalgias), respiratory (URI and cough), and gastrointestinal (diarrhea, abdominal pain, and nausea/vomiting) [18].

No conclusions can be drawn for the long-term (greater than 1 year) use of SPB. Also, the safety profile produced is characteristic of this specific extract, which, as discussed, was examined for relative uniformity with the majority of available extracts on the market but by no means all of them (see section on product variability).

Adverse effects examined in the Cochrane review also concluded them to be generally mild. When compared to placebo, no treatment arm reported an incidence greater than 5%, and none of the comparisons were statistically significant [12].

Like pharmaceutical agents, large-scale phase IV clinical trials would be needed to adequately assess for safety.

In conclusion, lifestyle modification can provide some mild benefit for nocturia. It is uncertain if any of the nutraceutical products can provide any improvement greater than placebo in reducing nocturia.

References

1. Lowe FC, Fagelman E. Phytotherapy in the treatment of benign prostatic hyperplasia: an update. Urology. 1999;53(4):671–8.
2. Bales GT, Christiano AP, Kirsh EJ, Gerber GS. Phytotherapeutic agents in the treatment of lower urinary tract symptoms: a demographic analysis of awareness and use at the University of Chicago. Urology. 1999;54(1):86–9.
3. Buck AC. Is there a scientific basis for the therapeutic effects of serenoa repens in benign prostatic hyperplasia? Mechanisms of action. J Urol. 2004;172(5 Pt 1):1792–9.
4. Levin RM, Hass MA, Bellamy F, Horan P, Whitbeck K, Chow PH, et al. Effect of oral Tadenan treatment on rabbit bladder structure and function after partial outlet obstruction. J Urol. 2002;167(5):2253–9.
5. Levin RM, Whitbeck C, Horan P, Bellamy F. Low-dose tadenan protects the rabbit bladder from bilateral ischemia/reperfusion-induced contractile dysfunction. Phytomedicine. 2005;12(1–2):17–24.
6. Feifer AH, Fleshner NE, Klotz L. Analytical accuracy and reliability of commonly used nutritional supplements in prostate disease. J Urol. 2002;168(1):150–4. discussion 4.

7. Habib FK, Wyllie MG. Not all brands are created equal: a comparison of selected components of different brands of Serenoa repens extract. Prostate Cancer Prostatic Dis. 2004;7(3):195–200.
8. Wilt TJ, Ishani A, Stark G, MacDonald R, Lau J, Mulrow C. Saw palmetto extracts for treatment of benign prostatic hyperplasia: a systematic review. JAMA. 1998;280(18):1604–9.
9. Boyle P, Robertson C, Lowe F, Roehrborn C. Updated meta-analysis of clinical trials of Serenoa repens extract in the treatment of symptomatic benign prostatic hyperplasia. BJU Int. 2004;93(6):751–6.
10. Willetts KE, Clements MS, Champion S, Ehsman S, Eden JA. Serenoa repens extract for benign prostate hyperplasia: a randomized controlled trial. BJU Int. 2003;92(3):267–70.
11. Bent S, Kane C, Shinohara K, Neuhaus J, Hudes ES, Goldberg H, et al. Saw palmetto for benign prostatic hyperplasia. N Engl J Med. 2006;354(6):557–66.
12. Tacklind J, MacDonald R, Rutks I, Wilt TJ. Serenoa repens for benign prostatic hyperplasia. Cochrane Database Syst Rev. 2009;15(2):CD001423.
13. Ishani A, MacDonald R, Nelson D, Rutks I, Wilt TJ. Pygeum africanum for the treatment of patients with benign prostatic hyperplasia: a systematic review and quantitative meta-analysis. Am J Med. 2000;109(8):654–64.
14. Carraro JC, Raynaud JP, Koch G, Chisholm GD, Di Silverio F, Teillac P, et al. Comparison of phytotherapy (Permixon) with finasteride in the treatment of benign prostate hyperplasia: a randomized international study of 1,098 patients. Prostate. 1996;29(4):231–40. discussion 41–2.
15. Debruyne F, Koch G, Boyle P, Da Silva FC, Gillenwater JG, Hamdy FC, et al. Comparison of a phytotherapeutic agent (Permixon) with an alpha-blocker (Tamsulosin) in the treatment of benign prostatic hyperplasia: a 1-year randomized international study. Prog Urol. 2002;12(3):384–92. discussion 94–4.
16. Debruyne F, Boyle P, Calais Da Silva F, Gillenwater JG, Hamdy FC, Perrin P, et al. Evaluation of the clinical benefit of permixon and tamsulosin in severe BPH patients-PERMAL study subset analysis. Eur Urol. 2004;45(6):773–9. discussion 9–80.
17. Hizli F, Uygur MC. A prospective study of the efficacy of Serenoa repens, tamsulosin, and Serenoa repens plus tamsulosin treatment for patients with benign prostate hyperplasia. Int Urol Nephrol. 2007;39(3):879–86.
18. Avins AL, Bent S, Staccone S, Badua E, Padula A, Goldberg H, et al. A detailed safety assessment of a saw palmetto extract. Complement Ther Med. 2008;16(3):147–54.

Chapter 12
Nocturia: Proposals for Future Investigation

Jeffrey P. Weiss

Keywords Nocturia • Future investigation • Frequency–volume charts
• Questionnaires • Health economics • Near nocturia • Outcomes of therapy

Nocturia is an entity whose clinical, pathological, and therapeutic features are currently being shaped. Further research is necessary to help separate nocturia from its historical "bundling" with other LUTS. For example, suggestions in popular media that overactive bladder and prostate therapies are capable of achieving clinically meaningful improvements in nocturia remain to be verified.

Nocturia investigations should be carried out utilizing both frequency–volume charts and validated questionnaires capturing QoL and bother related specifically to nocturia. The following are proposals for potential future investigation related to nocturia:

- Validation and clarification of the definitions of both nocturia (with regard to any night awakening owing to the desire to pass urine, the ICS definition, versus the more clinically bothersome nocturia × 2–3 or more), nocturnal polyuria cut points (see Chap. 4), and diminished nocturnal bladder capacity [1, 2]. It would be beneficial (for the purpose of targeted therapy) to better characterize diminished nocturnal bladder capacity as resulting from either nocturnal detrusor overactivity or abnormal nocturnal triggering of bladder and/or urethral sensations.
- Basic research into the following areas of interest: age-related circadian rhythms, the effects of "near nocturia" (nocturnal arousals due to the sensation of needing to pass urine, followed by sleep without voiding) on sleep quality, [3] the question of whether patients are voiding because they are awakened by the need to

---

J.P. Weiss, MD, FACS (✉)
Department of Urology, SUNY Downstate College of Medicine,
VA New York Harbor Healthcare System, Brooklyn, NY, USA
e-mail: urojock@aol.com

void, or are voiding because they are awakened by something else (i.e., insomnia), and whether, upon such awakenings, they void with little or no desire.
- Research to determine the extent to which nocturia interferes with objectively (polysomnographically) assessed sleep duration and sleep continuity, with particular emphasis on the duration of sleep prior to the first awakening of the night and the relative amount of slow wave sleep that occurs during that period.
- Epidemiological research regarding studies of nocturia involving the following aspects: prevalence, incidence/natural history, bother, effect on quality of life and effect on mortality in different age categories, gender, and worldwide populations. Considerable information may be gleaned by accessing baseline characteristics of populations of patients with severe nocturia and outcomes of nocturia therapeutic trials as gathered by various elements of the pharmaceutical industry.
- Patient-reported outcome research into the most relevant endpoints to consider in research (e.g., number of nocturia episodes, nocturia-related impairment in QoL, nocturia-related impairment of sleep quality, morbidity, mortality, and clinically significant improvement)?
- Health economics research into the true costs of nocturia to society and the individual, as well as the impact and cost effectiveness of different therapeutic strategies at both patient and systems levels. Study the relationship between bother from nocturia and the individual's employment status.
- Outcomes of therapy for nocturia (e.g., behavioral; timed diuretics; timed antidiuretics; antimuscarinics; lower urinary tract surgery for obstruction, overactive or underactive bladders; continuous positive airway pressure for sleep apneics; and combinations of therapies) in clinical practice.
- Address the question as to whether antidiuretic therapy should be limited to patients with diary-confirmed NP and whether antimuscarinic therapy is effective in subpopulations of patients with significant nocturnal urgency [4, 5].
- The relationships between nocturia and obesity, fluid and sodium intake, cardiovascular and renal disease.

Finally, a goal for determining the effects of multiple incremental therapies for nocturia appears to be sensible in view of the well-known multifactorial nature of its etiology. Algorithms for both initial (i.e., empiric) and subsequent (e.g., cause-specific) management of various groups such as the young working population, frail elderly, and men versus women would seem to be desirable.

References

1. Tikkinen KA, Johnson 2nd TM, Tammela TL, et al. Nocturia frequency, bother, and quality of life: how often is too often? A population-based study in Finland. Eur Urol. 2010;57:488–96.
2. Burton C, Parsons M, Weiss JP, Coats A. Reference values for the nocturnal bladder capacity index. Neurourol Urodyn. 2011;30:52–7.

3. Stanley N. The physiology of sleep and the impact of ageing. Eur Urol. 2005;3:17–23.
4. Rackley R, Weiss JP, Rovner ES, Wang JT, Guan Z. Nighttime dosing with tolterodine reduces bladder-related nocturnal micturitions in patients with overactive bladder and nocturia. Urology. 2006;67:731–6.
5. Brubaker L, Fitzgerald MP. Nocturnal polyuria and nocturia relief in patients treated with solifenacin for overactive bladder symptoms. Int Urogynecol J. 2007;18:737–41.

Index

A
Age factors, 13–14
American Urologic Association Symptom score (AUASS), 112, 116
Antidiuretic pharmacotherapy
  arginine vasopressin (AVP), 136–138
  desmopressin
    Noctopus trials, 138–141
    structure and mechanism of action, 137–138
    USA and Canada trial, 141–142
  hyponatremia, 142
Antidiuretic therapy, 7
Antimuscarinics, 128, 133
Antimuscarinictherapy, overactive bladder, 128–130
Arginine vasopressin (AVP), 136–138

B
Benign prostatic hyperplasia (BPH), 77, 89–91, 95, 96, 115–124
BMI, 29–30

C
Cardiovascular diseases, 19–21
Combined therapy, 132
Comorbid disease, 151, 158
Coronary disease, 91–92

D
Depression, 90–91
Desmopressin, 127
  Noctopus trials, 138–141
  structure and mechanism of action, 137–138
  USA and Canada trial, 141–142
Detrusor overactivity, 111, 112
Diabetes, 94
Diabetes insipidus, 4
Diary-based population analysis
  frequency volume charts (FVC), 60–61
  Krimpen study protocol
    baseline round, 61–65
    cross-sectional data, 66–70
    follow-up rounds, 65
    longitudinal data, 70–74

E
Elderly
  causes, 148, 149
  diary-based population analysis (*see* Diary-based population analysis)
  family and caregiver burden, 150
  healthcare costs, 150
  morbidity, 151
  mortality, 152
  quality-of-life impact, 148–149
  sleep disturbance, 150
  treatment issues, 152–153
Ethnicity, 15

F
Falls, 48, 89, 151
Family and caregiver burden, 150
Female reproductive/gynecologic factors, 27–28
Fesoterodine, 129, 130
Finasteride, 161

Finnish National Nocturia and Overactive Bladder (FINNO), 79, 86–89, 91–95, 97, 98
Fluid volume disturbance, 24–26
Fractures, 48, 89
Frequency volume charts (FVC), 60–61

G
Gender factors, 15
Global polyuria, 4–6, 24–25
Gravidity, 97–98

H
Healthcare costs, 150
Health economics research, 166
Herbal/dietary supplements
    difficulties in evaluation, 159–160
    efficacy, 160–161
    finasteride, 161
    Permixon®, 161–162
    plant extracts/supplements, 158
    product variability, 160
    Saw palmetto berry (SPB) mechanisms of action, 159
    Saw palmetto for treatment of enlarged prostates (STEP) trial, 162
    side effects monitoring, 163
    tamsulosin, 161–162
Hormone therapy, 98
Hours of uninterrupted sleep (HUS), 120, 123
Hypertension, 91–92
Hyponatremia, 142

I
Incidence, 81–85
International Consultation on Incontinence Modular Questionnaire–Nocturia Quality of Life questionnaire, 86
International Consultation on Incontinence Nocturia Quality of Life (NQOL), 118–120, 123
International Consultation on Incontinence Questionnaire for Nocturia (ICIQ-N), 5
International Prostate Symptom Score (IPSS), 60, 61, 64, 67, 73, 74

K
Krimpen study protocol
    baseline round, 61–65
    cross-sectional data, 66–70
    follow-up rounds, 65
    longitudinal data
        nocturia prevalence, 70
        nocturnal polyuria prevalence, 70–74

L
Latchkey syndrome, 113
Lifestyle and behavioral factors, 28–29, 96
Lifestyle changes, 157–158
Lower urinary tract factors, 16–19
Lower urinary tract pharmacotherapy
    antimuscarinic therapy, overactive bladder, 128–130
    combined therapy, 132
    obstructive BPH management therapy, 130–132
    others, 132–133
Lower urinary tract symptoms (LUTS), 77, 79, 85, 89, 90, 95–97, 115, 116, 120–124, 147, 149, 150

M
Maximum voided volume (MVV), 2
Medical conditions
    BMI and obesity, 29–30
    cardiovascular diseases, 19–21
    conditions
        benign prostatic hyperplasia, 89–90
        depression, 90–91
        hypertension and coronary disease, 91–92
        neurological diseases, 93
        nocturnal polyuria, 93–94
        obesity and diabetes, 94
        overactive bladder and detrusor overactivity, 94–95
        prostate cancer, 95–96
    demographic factors
        age, 13–14
        ethnic or cultural groups, 15
        gender, 15
    female reproductive/gynecologic factors, 27–28
    fluid intake, 30–31
    fluid volume disturbance, 24–26
    lifestyle and behavioral factors, 28–29, 96
    lower urinary tract factors, 16–19
    physical activity, 31–32
    pulmonary, 21–22
    race/ethnicity and socioeconomic status, 96–97
    reproductive factors in women
        gravidity/pregnancy, parity and post-partum period, 97–98

Index

menopause and hormone therapy, 98
pelvic surgery, 98
sleep-related factors, 22–24
smoking, 31
socioeconomic factors, 26–27
Menopause, 98
Micturition, 110
Minimally invasive surgical therapies (MIST), 122
Mixed nocturia, 4
Morbidity, 37–38, 151
Mortality, 37–38, 89, 152

N
Near nocturia, 165
Neurological diseases, 93
Nighttime falls. *See* Falls
Noctopus trials, 138–141
Nocturia
  antidiuretic pharmacotherapy (*see* Antidiuretic pharmacotherapy)
  consequences, 6
  definition, 1–2, 111–112
  diary-based classification
    decreased nocturnal bladder capacity, 3–4
    global polyuria, 4–6
    vs. medical conditions, 3
    mixed nocturia, 4
    nocturnal polyuria (NP), 2–3
    nocturnal urine volume (NUV), 2
  diary-based population analysis (*see* Diary-based population analysis)
  frequency–volume charts, 165
  future investigation, 165–166
  impact
    bother and quality of life, 85–88
    falls, fractures and mortality, 89
  lower urinary tract pharmacotherapy (*see* Lower urinary tract pharmacotherapy)
  older persons (*see* Elderly)
  vs. overactive bladder, 112–113
  predictors and risk factors (*see* Medical conditions)
  sleep deprivation, 6–7 (*see also* Sleep; Sleep apnea; Sleep disorders)
  therapy, 7–8
  treatment with alternative therapies
    lifestyle changes, 157–158
    supplements, 158–162 (*see also* Herbal/dietary supplements)
Nocturia Nocturnal Enuresis and Sleep-interruption Questionnaire (NNES-Q), 148
Nocturia Quality-of-Life (N-QOL), 5
Nocturnal polyuria (NP), 2–3, 62, 65, 68, 72, 93–94, 136–144
Nocturnal urine volume (NUV), 2, 25–26

O
Obesity, 29–30, 94
Obstructive BPH management therapy, 130–132
Obstructive sleep apnea (OSA), 161. *See also* Sleep apnea
Older persons. *See* Elderly
Overactive bladder (OAB)
  antidiuretic pharmacotherapy, 136, 137, 140–143
  antimuscarinic therapy, 128–130
  definition, 110–111
  and detrusor overactivity, 94–95
  future research, 113
  vs. nocturia, 112–113

P
Parity, 97–98
Pelvic surgery, 98
Permixon®, 160–162
Physical activity, 31–32
Pittsburgh Sleep Quality Index (PSQI), 5
Plant extracts/supplements, 158
Poor sleep, 48, 52
Post-partum period, 97–98
Predictors and risk factors. *See* Medical conditions
Pregnancy, 97–98
Prescribing cascade, 152
Prevalence, 79–81
Prostate cancer, 95–96
  treatment (*see* Surgical treatment)
Pulmonary diseases, 21–22

Q
Quality-of-life (QoL), 85–88, 148–149

R
Race/ethnicity and socioeconomic status, 96–97
Radical prostatectomy (RP), 121
Reproductive factors in women
  gravidity/pregnancy, parity and post-partum period, 97–98
  menopause and hormone therapy, 98
  pelvic surgery, 98
Risk factors. *See* Medical conditions

S

Saw palmetto berry (SPB) mechanisms of action, 159
Saw palmetto for treatment of enlarged prostates (STEP) trial, 162, 163
Sleep
 continuity, 46–48
 disturbance, 52, 150
 duration
  in people with nocturia *versus* controls, 42
  quantity, 39–42
 efficiency, 43, 46
 stages, 42
 SWS, 43–45
Sleep apnea
 acute and intermediary mechanisms, 50
 clinical syndrome, 49
 diagnosis and treatment, 50–52
 nocturia-related sleep deprivation, 52–53
Sleep disorders
 day time functioning and quality of life (QoL), 38–39
 falls and fractures, 48
 medical conditions, 22–24
 morbidity and mortality, 37–38
Sleep-related factors, 22–24
Smoking, 31
Socioeconomic factors, 26–27
Solifenacin, 128, 129

Surgical treatment
 in men with BPH and nocturia
  BPH impact index, 116, 118
  HUS, 120
  IPSS/AUASS, 116, 117
  NQOL, 118–120
 therapy
  effect of PVP laser, 122–123
  minimally invasive surgical therapies (MIST), 122
  radical prostatectomy (RP), 121
  regression analysis and NQOL, 123
  transurethral resection of the prostate (TURP), 121–122

T

Tamsulosin, 161–162
Tolterodine, 129, 130, 132
Transurethral resection prostate (TURP), 7, 115, 121–123
Trospium chloride, 129

U

Uncontrolled diabetes mellitus, 4
Urgency, 110, 112, 113
Urgency Perception Score, 110–111
USA and Canada trial, 141–142

W

Water deprivation testing, 5